THE MEDITERRA[N] DIET COOKE[BOOK]

THE COMPLETE DASH DIET COOKING GUIDE FOR BEGINNERS TO LOWER BLOOD PRESSURE WITH 21-DAY WITH QUICK AND EASY LOW SODIUM RECIPES

Claudia Rivera

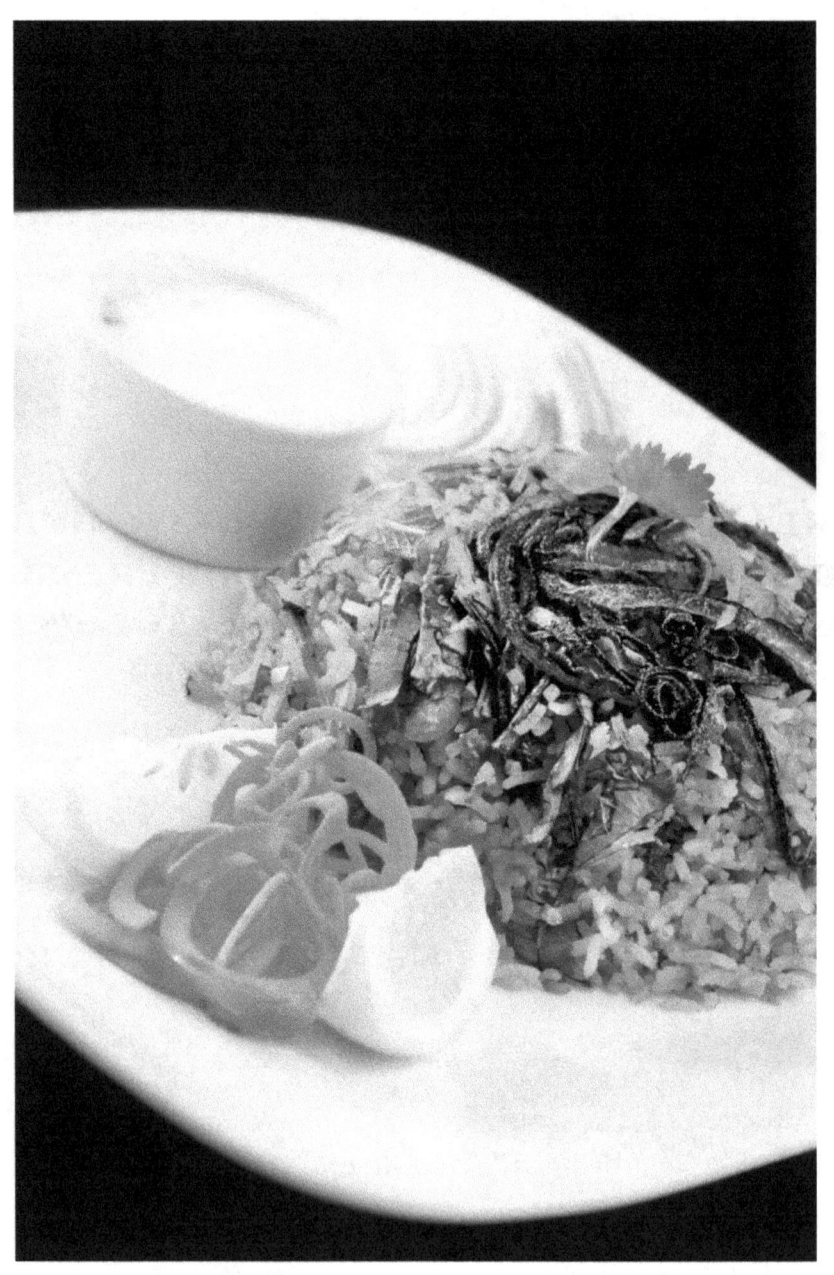

© Copyright 2020 by Claudia Rivera - All rights reserved.

The following Book is reproduced below with the goal of providing information that is as accurate and reliable as possible. Regardless, purchasing this Book can be seen as consent to the fact that both the publisher and the author of this book are in no way experts on the topics discussed within and that any recommendations or suggestions that are made herein are for entertainment purposes only. Professionals should be consulted as needed prior to undertaking any of the action endorsed herein.

This declaration is deemed fair and valid by both the American Bar Association and the Committee of Publishers Association and is legally binding throughout the United States.

Furthermore, the transmission, duplication, or reproduction of any of the following work including specific information will be considered an illegal act irrespective of if it is done electronically or in print. This extends to creating a secondary or tertiary copy of the work or a recorded copy and is only allowed with the express written consent from the Publisher. All additional right reserved.

The information in the following pages is broadly considered a truthful and accurate account of facts and as such, any inattention, use, or misuse of the information in question by the reader will render any resulting actions solely under their purview. There are no scenarios in which the publisher or the original author of this work can be in any fashion deemed liable for any hardship or damages that may befall them after undertaking information described herein.

Additionally, the information in the following pages is intended only for informational purposes and should thus be thought of as universal. As befitting its nature, it is presented without assurance regarding its prolonged validity or interim quality. Trademarks that are mentioned are done without written consent and can in no way be considered an endorsement from the trademark holder.

WHAT IS DASH DIET ?

DASH stands for Dietary Approaches to Stop Hypertension. The DASH diet is a lifelong approach to healthy eating that's designed to help treat or prevent high blood pressure (hypertension).The DASH diet emphasizes vegetables, fruits and low-fat dairy foods and moderate amounts of whole grains, fish, poultry and nuts.
DASH may also affect other areas of health (Decreases cancer risk ,Lowers metabolic syndrome risk, Lowers diabetes risk, Decreases heart disease risk.)

The DASH Program :

Grains: 5 daily servings
Vegetables: 3 daily servings
Fruits: 4 daily servings
Low-fat or fat-free dairy products: 2 daily servings
Meat, poultry, and fish: 2 or less daily servings
So, you can pick and choose your favorite meals and enjoy them at any time of the day, from dawn to dusk.
You shouldn't expect DASH to help you shed weight on its own as it was designed fundamentally to lower blood pressure. Weight loss may simply be an added perk.

Look Inside

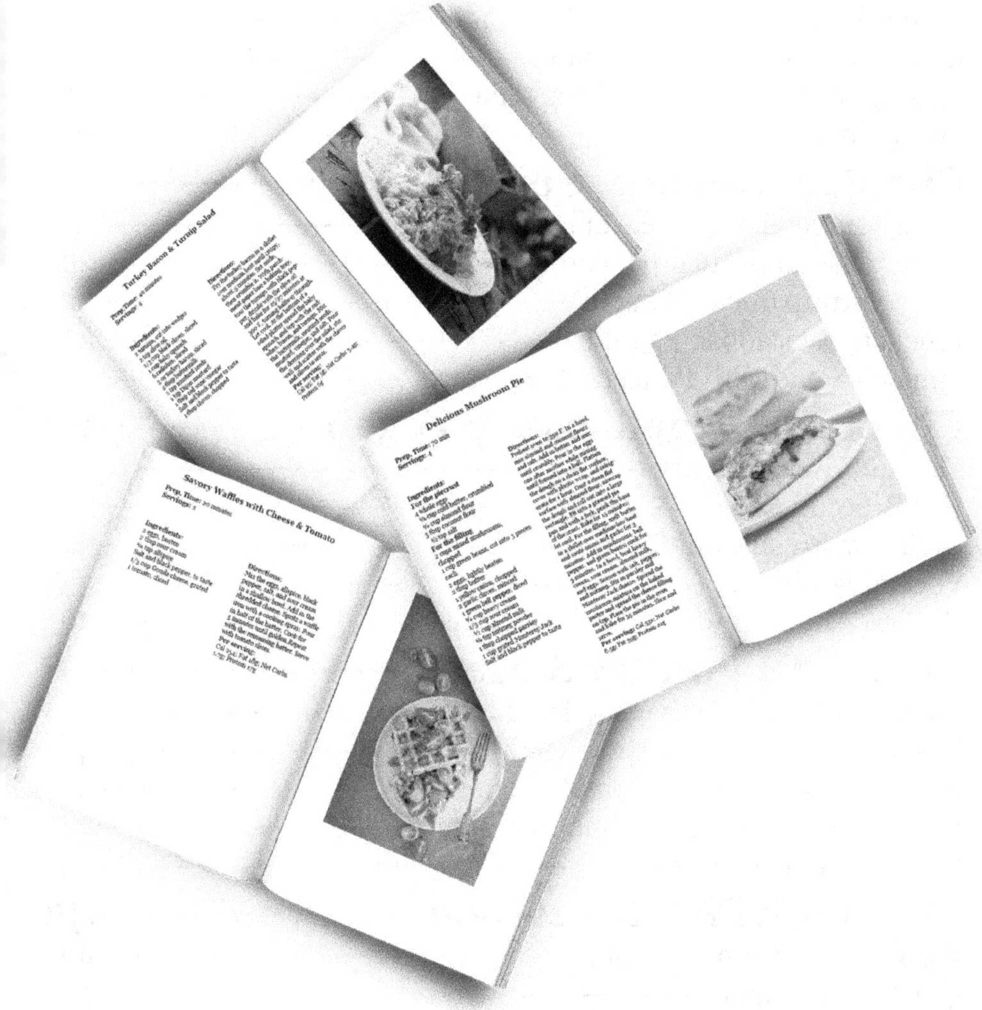

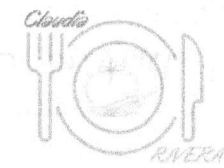

Table of Contents

Chapter 1 Breakfast — 8
Ham & Cheese Keto Sandwiches — 9
Savory Waffles with Cheese & Tomato — 10
Zesty Zucchini Bread with Nuts — 12
Bacon, Cheese & Avocado Mug Cakes — 14
Pumpkin & Zucchini Bread — 16

Chapter 2 Salads, Soups & Stews — 18
Mediterranean Artichoke Salad — 19
Turkey Bacon & Turnip Salad — 20
Fiery Shrimp Cocktail Salad — 22
Chicken, Avocado & Egg Bowls — 24
Spinach Salad with Pancetta & Mustard — 26

Chapter 3 Vegetarian & Vegan — 28
Coconut Avocado Tart — 29
Hot Broccoli Rabe — 30
Delicious Mushroom Pie — 32
Vegetable Biryani — 34
Charred Broccoli with Tamarind Sauce — 36

Chapter 4 Poultry & Meat — 38
Citrus Pork with Cabbage & Tomatoes — 39
Baked Pork Sausage with Vegetables — 40
Pork Chops with Basil-Tomato Sauce — 42
Herb Pork Chops with Cranberry Sauce — 44
Barbecued Pork Chops — 46

Chapter 5 Fish & Seafood — 48
Parmesan Shrimp Scampi Pizza — 49
Quick Tuna Omelet — 50
Baked Haddock with Cheesy Topping — 52
Baked Cod with Parmesan and Almonds — 54
Greek Sea Bass with Olive Sauce — 56

Chapter 6 Snacks, Appetizers & Side Dishes — 58
Maple Tahini Straws — 59
Basil Spinach & Zucchini Lasagna — 60

Cauli Rice Arancini -- 62
Flaxseed Toasts with Avocado Paté --------------------------------- 64
Caramelized Onion & Cream Cheese Spread ---------------------- 66

Chapter 7 Desserts, Fruits & Drinks ------68
Chocolate Mousse Pots with Blackberries ------------------------- 69
Dark Chocolate Brownies --- 70
Favorite Peanut Butter Mousse ------------------------------------- 72
Avocado Mousse with Chocolate ------------------------------------ 74
Mascarpone Cream Mousse -- 76

Chapter 8 Lunch ------------------------------78
Marinara Turkey Linguine --- 79
Pasta Tortiglioni with Beef & Black Beans ------------------------ 80
Mustard Macaroni & Cheese -- 82
Green Goddess Mac 'n' Cheese ------------------------------------- 84
Chicken & Broccoli Fettuccine Alfredo ---------------------------- 86
Easy Brown Rice with Sunflower Seeds ---------------------------- 88
Spicy Linguine with Cherry Tomato & Basil ---------------------- 90

Chapter 9 Dinner -----------------------------92
Butternut Squash with Rice & Feta --------------------------------- 93
Avocado & Cherry Tomato Jasmine Rice -------------------------- 94
Date & Apple Risotto --- 95
Butternut Squash & Cheese Risotto -------------------------------- 97
Spring Risotto --- 99
Arroz con Pollo --- 101
Chicken & Broccoli Rice --- 103
Hawaiian Rice --- 105

CHAPTER 1 BREAKFAST

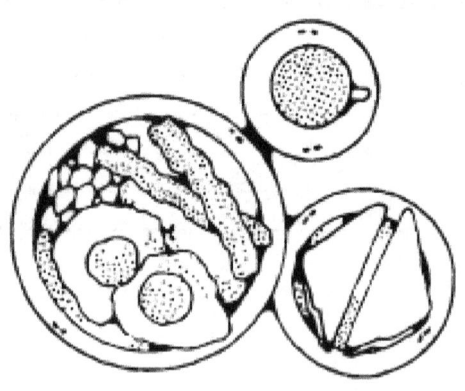

Ham & Cheese Keto Sandwiches

Prep. Time: 20 minutes
Servings: 2

Ingredients:
4 eggs
½ tsp baking powder
5 tbsp butter, softened
4 tbsp almond flour
2 tbsp psyllium husk powder
2 slices mozzarella cheese
2 slices smoked ham

Directions:
To make the buns, whisk together almond flour, baking powder, 4 tbsp of butter, husk powder, and eggs in a bowl; mix until a dough forms. Place the batter in two oven-proof mugs and microwave for 2 minutes or until firm. Remove, flip the buns over, cool, and cut in half. Put a slice of mozzarella cheese and a slice of ham on one bun half and top with the other. Warm the remaining butter in a skillet. Add sandwiches and grill until the cheese is melted. Serve and enjoy!

Per serving:
Cal 516; Fat 45g; Net Carbs 2.3g; Protein 23g

Savory Waffles with Cheese & Tomato

Prep. Time: 20 minutes
Servings: 2

Ingredients:
2 eggs, beaten
2 tbsp sour cream
¼ tsp allspice
Salt and black pepper, to taste
1/3 cup Gouda cheese, grated
1 tomato, sliced

Directions:
Mix the eggs, allspice, black pepper, salt, and sour cream in a shallow bowl. Add in the shredded cheese. Spritz a waffle iron with a cooking spray. Pour in half of the batter. Cook for 5 minutes until golden. Repeat with the remaining batter. Serve with tomato slices.

Per serving:
Cal 254; Fat 18g; Net Carbs 1.7g; Protein 17g

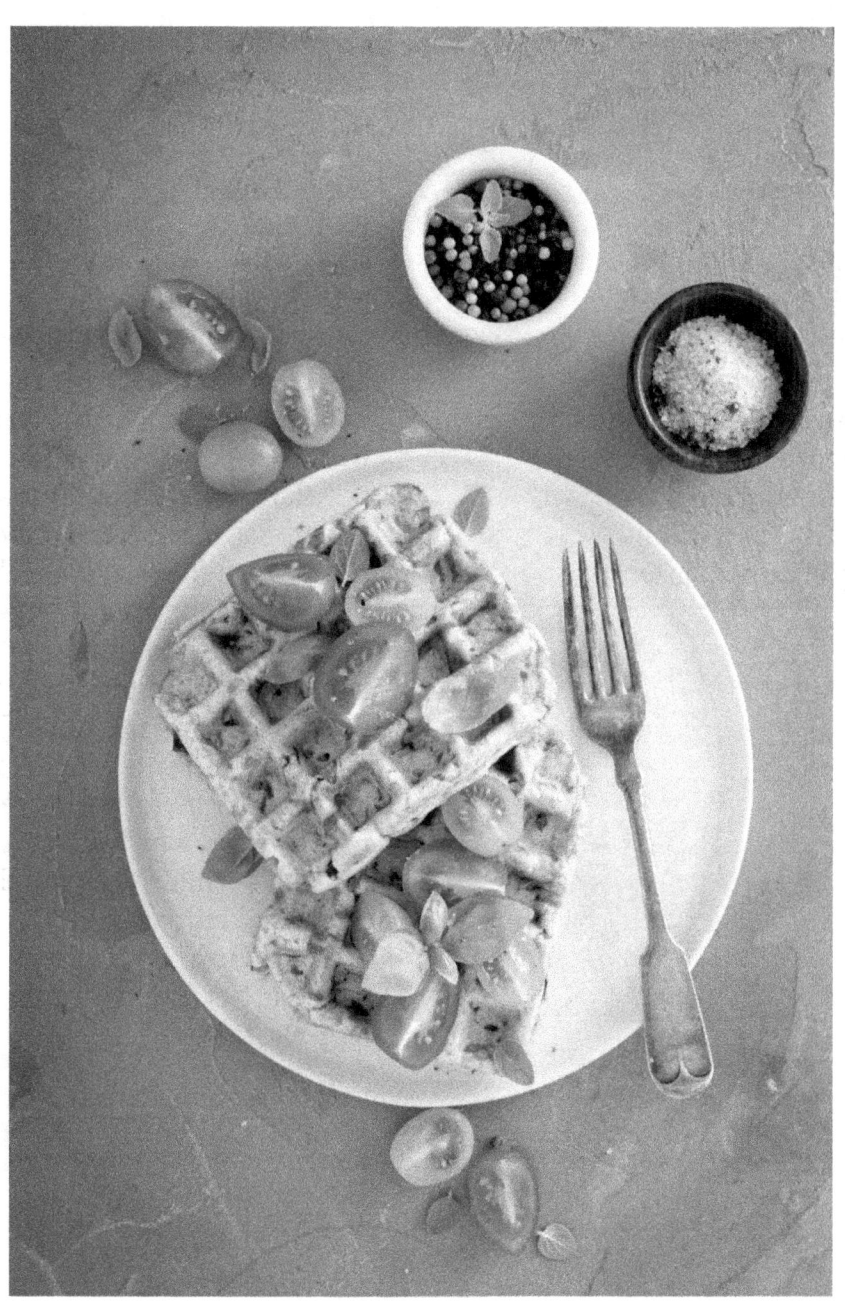

Zesty Zucchini Bread with Nuts

Prep. Time: 50 minutes
Servings: 4

Ingredients:
4 eggs
2/3 cup coconut flour
2 tsp baking powder
1 cup butter, softened
1 cup erythritol
2/3 cup ground almonds
1 lemon, zested and juiced
1 cup finely grated zucchini
1 cup whipped cream
1 tbsp chopped hazelnuts

Directions:
Preheat oven to 380 F. Grease a springform pan with and line with parchment paper. Set aside. In a bowl, beat the butter and erythritol until creamy and pale. Add eggs one after another while whisking. Add in baking powder and coconut flour and stir along with ground almonds, lemon zest, juice, and zucchini. Spoon the mixture into the pan. Bake for 40/42 minutes or until risen and a toothpick inserted into the cake comes out clean. Let cool inside the pan for 10 minutes. Transfer to a wire rack. Spread whipped cream on top and sprinkle with hazelnuts. Serve and enjoy!

Per serving:
Cal 781; Net Carbs 3.7g, Fat 69g, Protein 32g

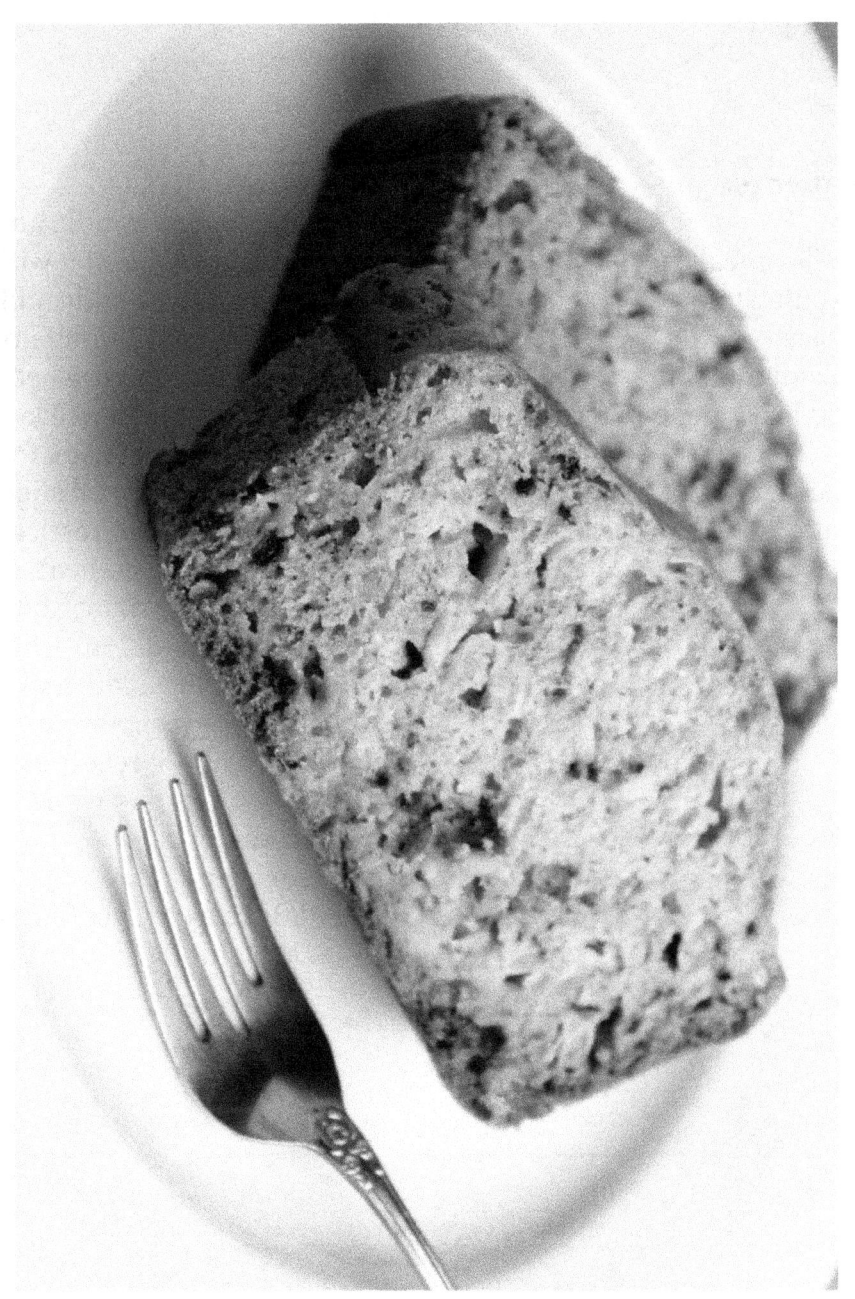

Bacon, Cheese & Avocado Mug Cakes

Prep. Time: 15 minutes
Servings: 2

Ingredients:
2 eggs
¼ cup flax meal
2 tbsp buttermilk
2 tbsp pesto
¼ cup almond flour
Salt and black pepper, to taste
2 tbsp ricotta cheese
2 oz bacon, sliced
1 avocado, sliced

Direction:
Whisk eggs, buttermilk, and pesto in a bowl. Season with salt and pepper. Gently add in flax meal and almond flour and divide the mixture between two greased ramekins. Place in the microwave and cook for 1-2 minutes. Leave to cool slightly before filling. In a nonstick skillet over medium heat, cook the bacon until crispy, about 5 minutes; set aside. Invert the ramekins onto a plate and cut in half, crosswise. Assemble the sandwiches by spreading ricotta cheese and topping with bacon and avocado slices.

Per serving:
Cal 488; Fat 37g; Net Carbs 3.9g; Protein 17g

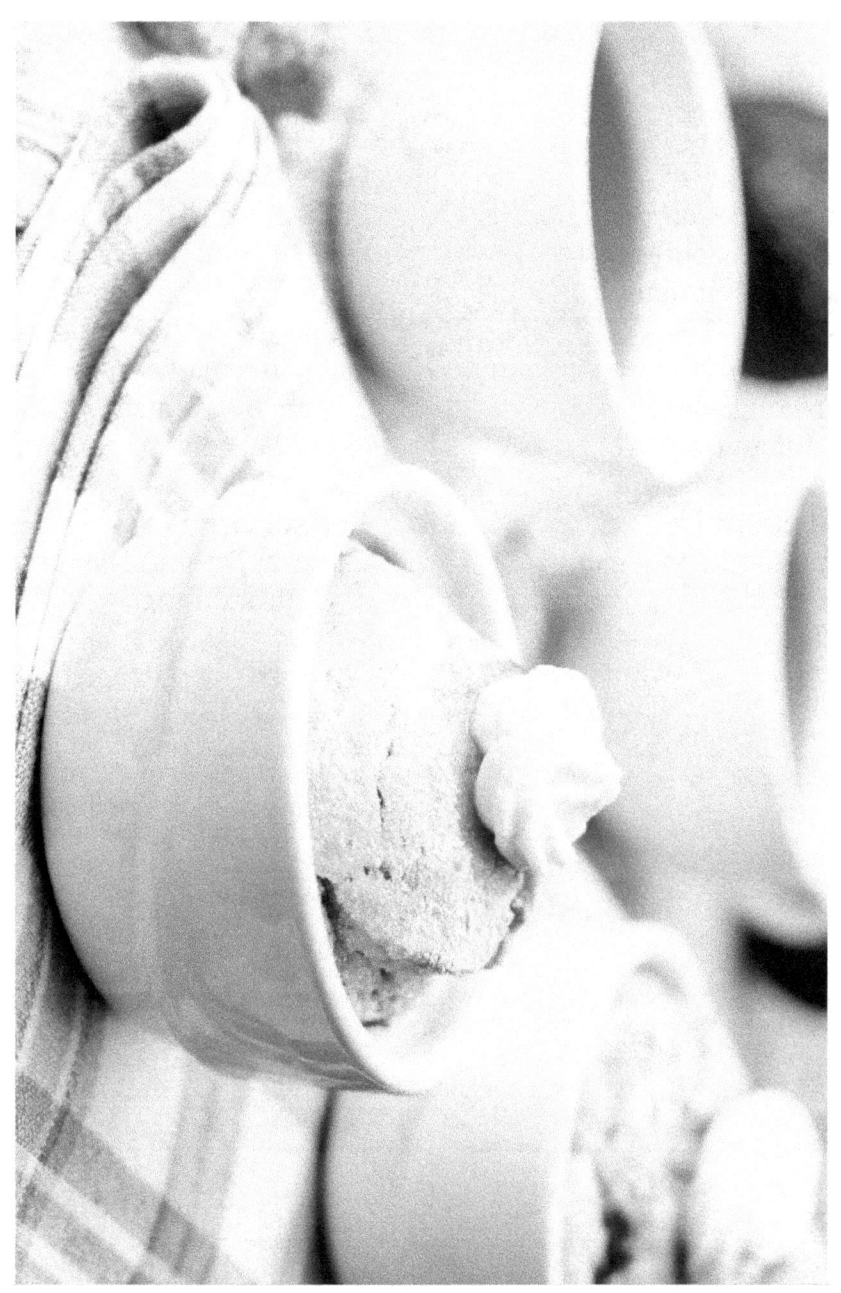

Pumpkin & Zucchini Bread

Prep. Time: 60 minutes
Servings: 4

Ingredients:
1 cup pumpkin, shredded
1 cup zucchini, shredded
1/3 cup coconut flour
6 eggs
1 tbsp olive oil
¾ tsp baking soda
1 tbsp cinnamon powder
½ tsp salt
½ cup buttermilk
1 tsp apple cider vinegar

Directions:
Preheat oven to 360 F. In a bowl, mix all the ingredients and stir to form a dough. Having poured batter into a greased loaf pan, bake for 45 minutes or until a toothpick comes out clean. Let cool for 5 minutes. Serve sliced.

Per serving:
Cal 202; Fat 12g; Net Carbs 4.5g; Protein 12g

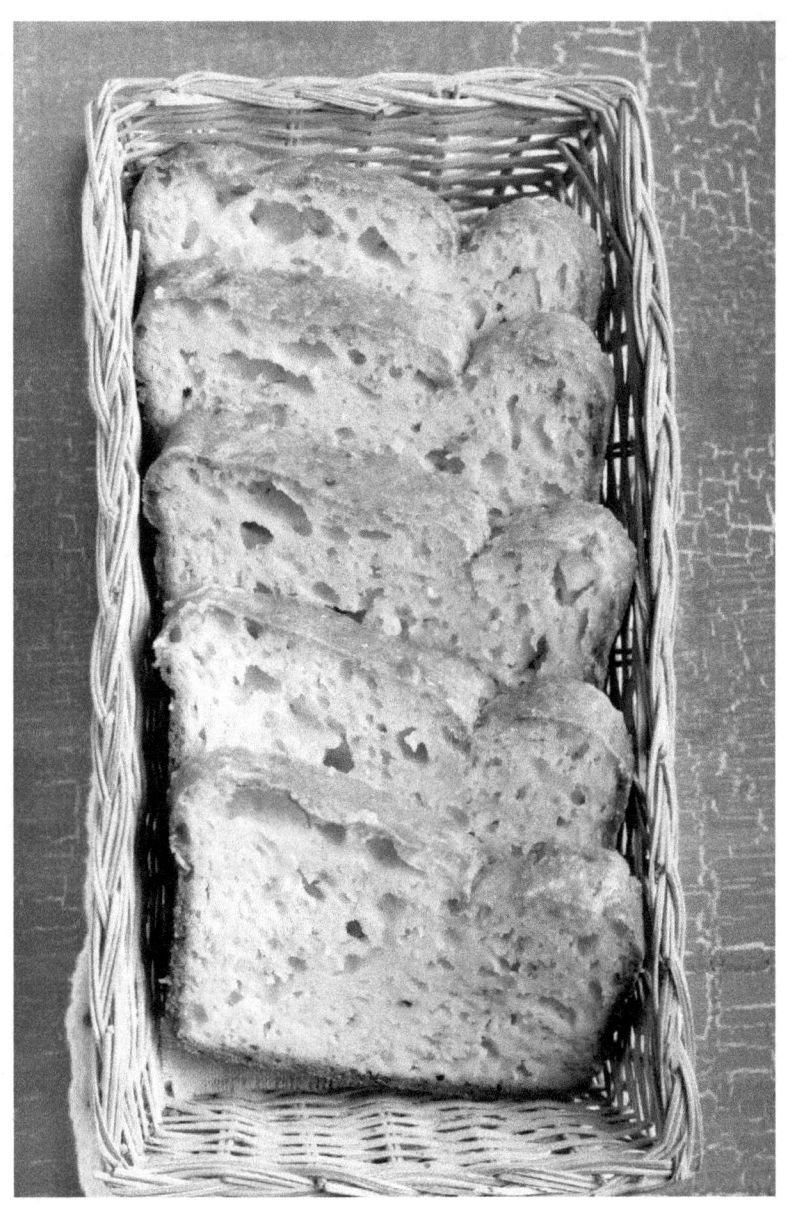

Chapter 2 Salads, Soups & Stews

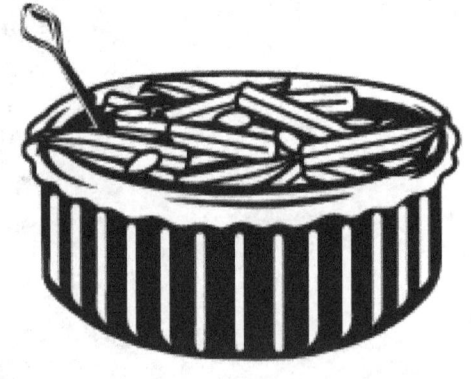

Mediterranean Artichoke Salad

Prep.Time: 30 minutes
Servings: 2

Ingredients:
6 baby artichoke hearts, halved
½ lemon, juiced
½ red onion, sliced
¼ cup cherry peppers, halved
¼ cup pitted olives, sliced
¼ cup olive oil
¼ tsp lemon zest
2 tsp balsamic vinegar
1 tbsp chopped dill
Salt and black pepper to taste
1 tbsp capers

Directions:
Boiling a pot of salted water. Add in the artichokes. Lower the heat and for 20 minutes let simmer until tender. Drain and place the artichokes in a small bowl to cool. Add in the rest of the ingredients, except for the olives; toss to combine well. Top with the olives and serve.

Per serving:
Cal 464; Fat 32g; Net Carbs 9.5g; Protein 13g

Turkey Bacon & Turnip Salad

Prep.Time: 40 minutes
Servings: 4

Ingredients:
2 turnips, cut into wedges
2 tsp olive oil
1/3 cup black olives, sliced
1 cup baby spinach
6 radishes, sliced
3 oz turkey bacon, sliced
4 tbsp buttermilk
2 tsp mustard seeds
1 tsp Dijon mustard
1 tbsp red wine vinegar
Salt and black pepper to taste
1 tbsp chives, chopped

Directions:
Fry the turkey bacon in a skillet over medium heat until crispy, about 5 minutes. Set aside, then crumble it. With parchment paper line a baking tray, toss the turnips with black pepper, drizzle with the olive oil and bake for 25/27 minutes at 390 F, turning halfway through. Let cool. At the bottom of a salad platter spread the baby spinach and top with the radishes, bacon, and turnips. Mix the buttermilk, mustard seeds, mustard, vinegar, and salt. Pour the dressing over the salad, stir well and scatter with the chives and olives to serve.

Per serving:
Cal 95; Fat 5g; Net Carbs 3.4g; Protein 6g

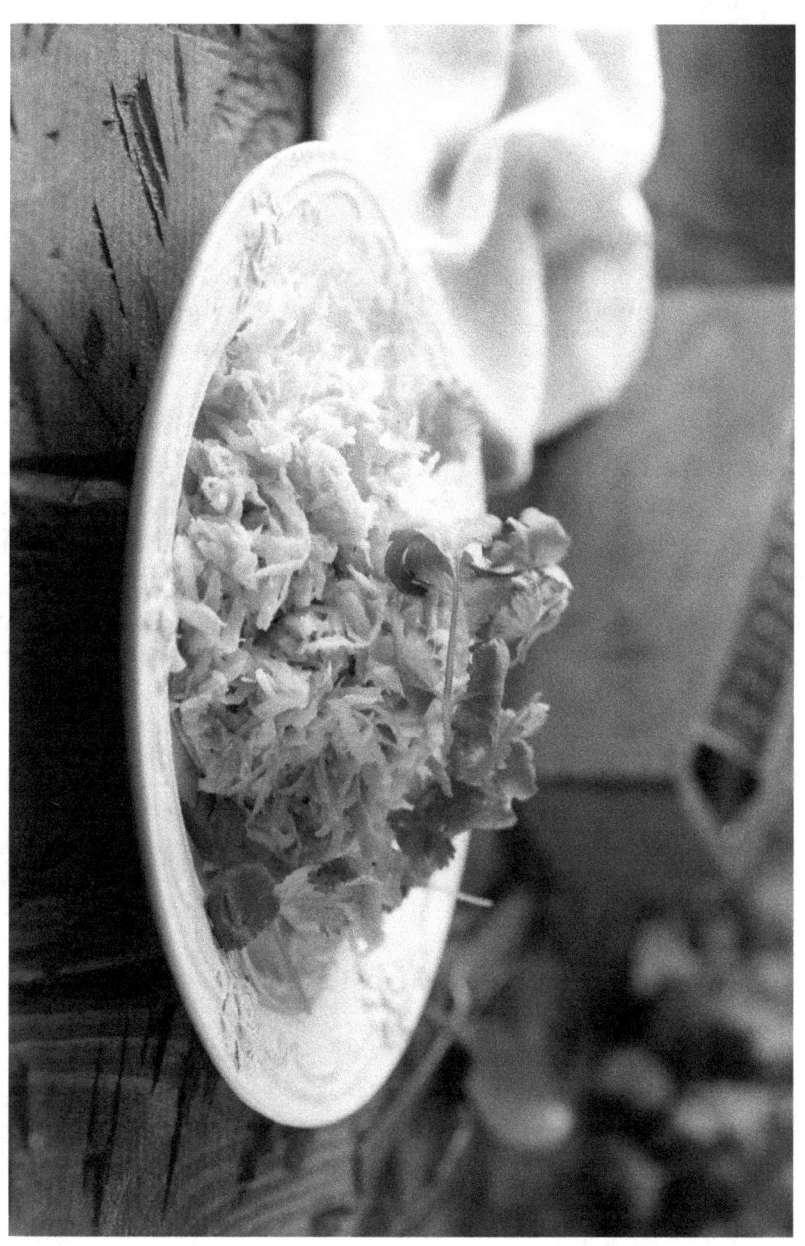

Fiery Shrimp Cocktail Salad

Prep.Time: 15 minutes
Servings: 4

Ingredients:
2 tbsp olive oil
½ head Romaine lettuce, torn
1 cucumber, cut into ribbons
½ lb shrimp, deveined
1 cup arugula
½ cup mayonnaise
2 tbsp Cholula hot sauce
½ tsp Worcestershire sauce
Salt and chili pepper to season
1 tbsp lemon juice
1 lemon, cut into wedges
4 dill weed

Directions:
Season the shrimp with salt and chili pepper. Warm the olive oil over medium heat and fry the shrimp for 3 minutes until pink and opaque. Set aside to cool. Place the mayonnaise, lemon juice, hot sauce, and Worcestershire sauce and mix until smooth and creamy in a bowl. Divide the lettuce and cucumber between 4 glass bowls. Top with shrimp and drizzle the hot dressing over. Scatter arugula on top and decorate with lemon wedges and dill to serve.

Per serving:
Cal 201; Fat 11g; Net Carbs 3.9g; Protein 14g

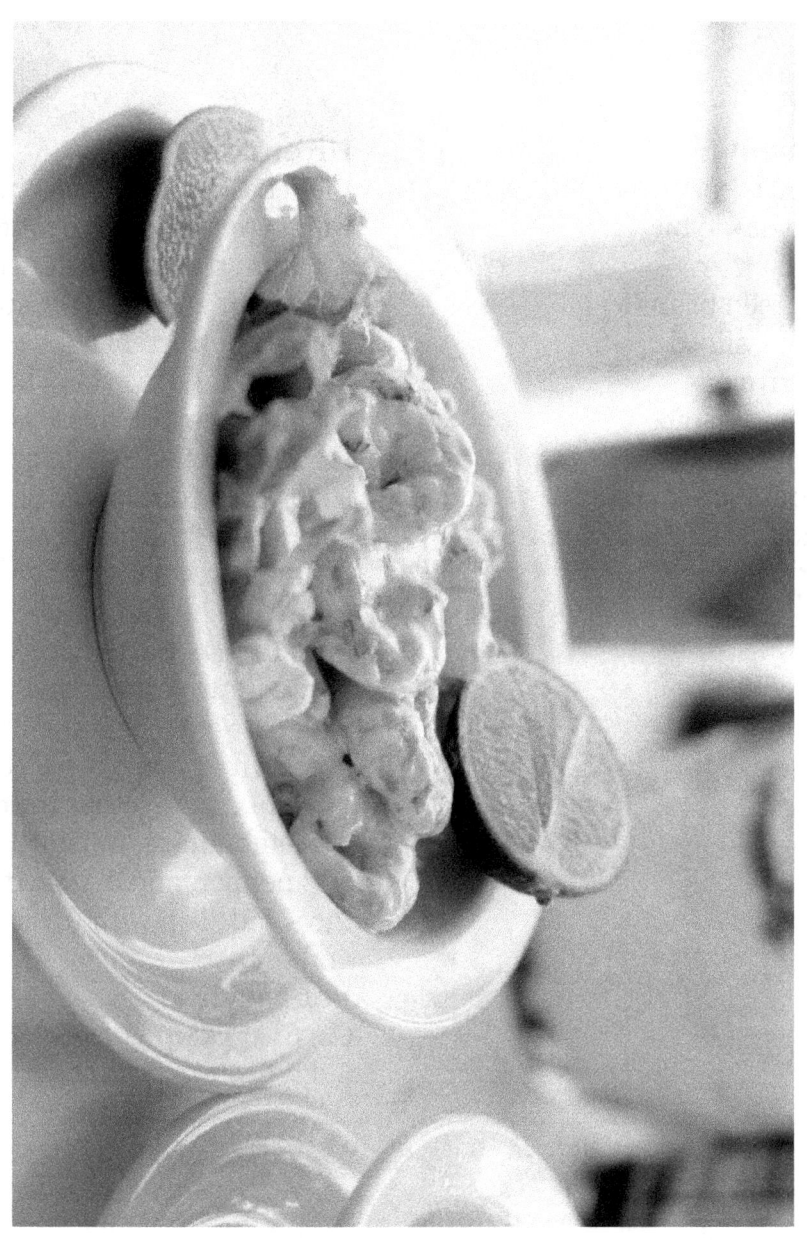

Chicken, Avocado & Egg Bowls

Prep.Time: 25 minutes
Servings: 2

Ingredients:
1 chicken breast, cubed
1 tbsp avocado oil
2 eggs
2 cups green beans
1 avocado, sliced
2 tbsp olive oil
2 tbsp lemon juice
1 tsp Dijon mustard
1 tbsp mint, chopped
Salt and black pepper to taste

Directions:
Blanch the green beans in salted water over medium heat for 4-5 minutes until the beans are bright green and crisp-tender. Refresh in cold water and drain. In the same boiling water, place the eggs and cook for 10 minutes. Remove to an ice bath to cool. Then, peel and slice them. Warm the avocado oil in a pan over medium heat. Cook the chicken for about 4 minutes. Divide the green beans between two salad bowls. Top with chicken, eggs, and avocado slices. In another bowl, combine mixing together the olive oil, lemon juice, mustard, salt, and pepper, and drizzle over the salad. Top with fresh mint and serve.

Per serving:
Cal 612; Fat 48g; Net Carbs 6.9g; Protein 27g

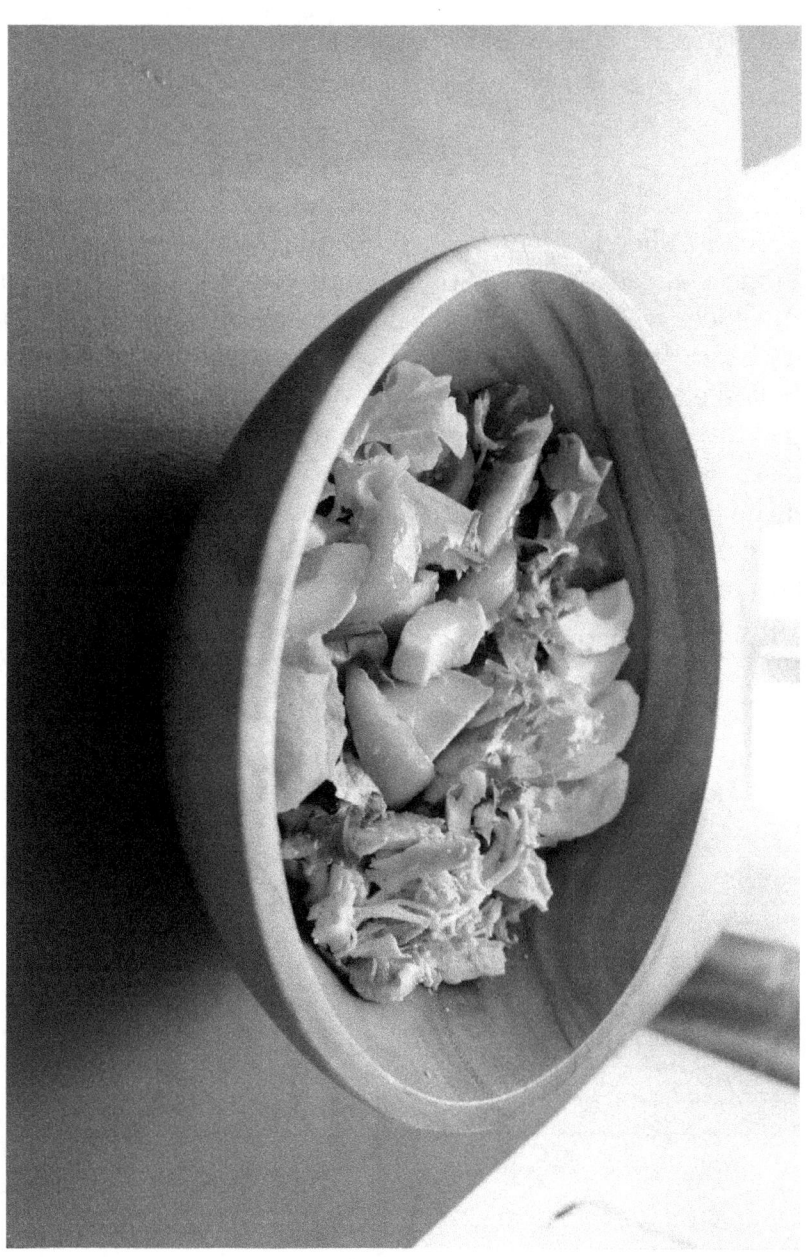

Spinach Salad with Pancetta & Mustard

Prep.Time: 20 minutes
Servings: 2

Ingredients:
1 cup spinach
1 large avocado, sliced
1 spring onion, sliced
2 pancetta slices
½ lettuce head, shredded
1 hard-boiled egg, chopped
Vinaigrette:
Salt to taste
¼ tsp garlic powder
3 tbsp olive oil
1 tsp Dijon mustard
1 tbsp white wine vinegar

Directions:
Chop the pancetta and fry in a skillet over medium heat for 5 minutes until crispy. Set aside to cool. Mix spinach, lettuce, egg, and spring onion in a bowl. Whisk the vinaigrette ingredients in another bowl. Pour the dressing over, toss to combine. Top with avocado and pancetta. Serve immediately.

Per serving:
Cal 547; Fat 51g; Net Carbs 4g; Protein 12g

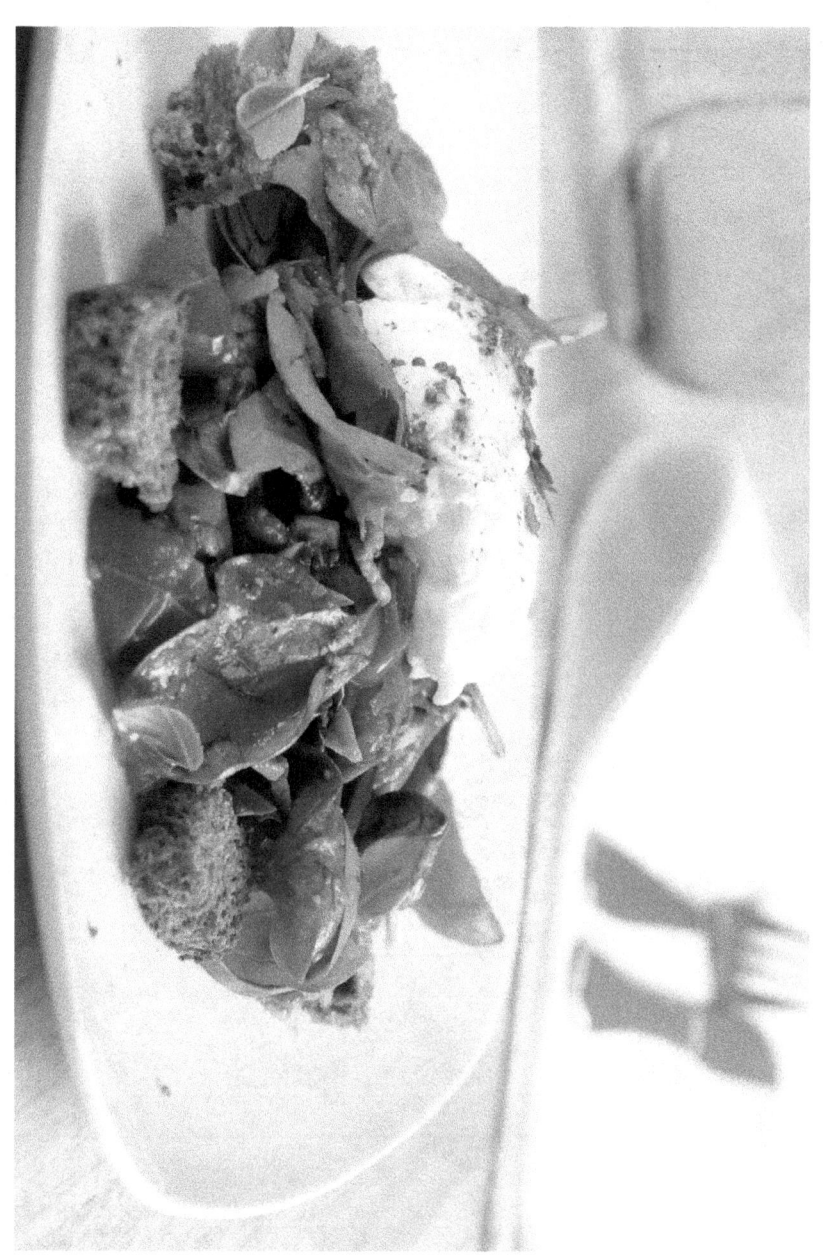

Chapter 3 Vegetarian & Vegan

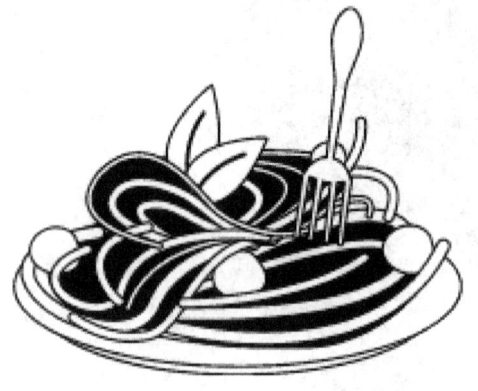

Coconut Avocado Tart

Prep. Time: 70 min
Servings: 4

Ingredients:
1¼ cups grated Parmesan
½ cup cream cheese
1 egg
4 tbsp coconut flour
4 tbsp chia seeds
¾ cup almond flour
1 tbsp psyllium husk powder
1 tsp baking powder
3 tbsp coconut oil
2 ripe avocados, mashed
1 cup mayonnaise
1 jalapeño pepper, minced
½ tsp onion powder
2 tbsp fresh parsley, chopped

Directions:
Preheat oven to 350 F. In a bowl, add coconut flour, chia seeds, almond flour, psyllium husk, baking powder, coconut oil, and 4 tbsp water. Blend until the resulting dough forms into a ball. Roll out dough on a springform pan lined with parchment paper. Bake for 15 minutes. In a bowl, put avocados, mayonnaise, egg, parsley, jalapeño pepper, onion powder, cream cheese, and Parmesan cheese; mix well. Remove the piecrust when ready and fill with the creamy mixture. Bake for 35-40 minutes until golden brown.

Per serving:
Cal 891; Net Carbs 10g; Fat 71g; Protein 24g

Hot Broccoli Rabe

Prep. Time: 15 min
Servings: 4

Ingredients:
1 tbsp olive oil
1 tbsp melted butter
1 lb broccoli rabe, trimmed
1 orange bell pepper, sliced
1 garlic clove, minced
1 tbsp red chili flakes
½ lemon, zested
2 tbsp cashew nuts, chopped
Salt and black pepper to taste

Directions:
Blanch broccoli in lightly salted water for 6-8 minutes or until tender; drain. Heat butter and olive oil in a skillet over medium heat and sauté garlic and bell pepper until softened, 5 minutes; season with salt and pepper. Toss in broccoli and lemon zest. Sprinkle with red chili flakes and chopped cashew. Serve and enjoy!

Per serving:
Cal 117; Net Carbs 1.7g; Fat 8.4g; Protein 3.7g

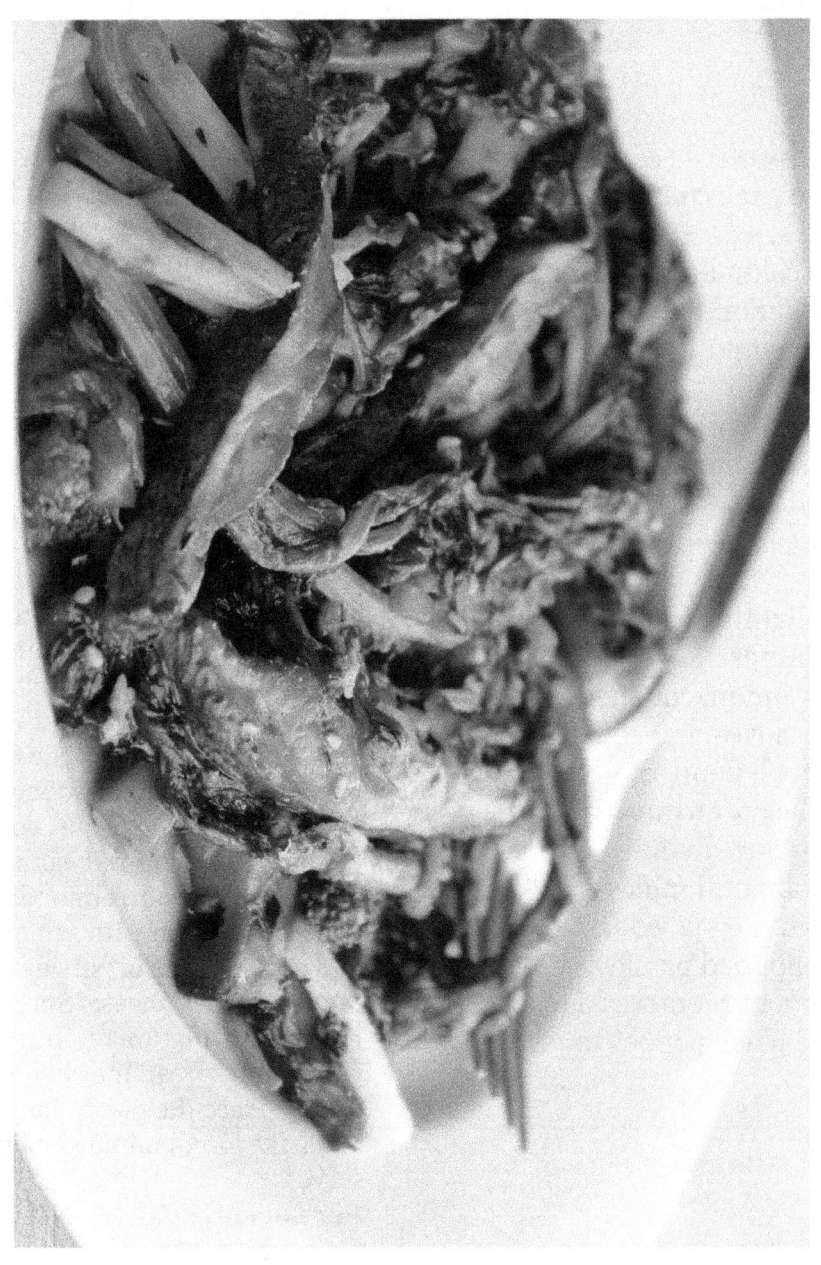

Delicious Mushroom Pie

Prep. Time: 70 min
Servings: 4

Ingredients:
For the piecrust
4 whole eggs
¼ cup cold butter, crumbled
¼ cup almond flour
3 tbsp coconut flour
½ tsp salt
For the filling
2 cups mixed mushrooms, chopped
1 cup green beans, cut into 3 pieces each
2 eggs, lightly beaten
2 tbsp butter
1 yellow onion, chopped
2 garlic cloves, minced
1 green bell pepper, diced
¼ cup heavy cream
1/3 cup sour cream
½ cup almond milk
¼ tsp nutmeg powder
1 tbsp chopped parsley
1 cup grated Monterey Jack
Salt and black pepper to taste

Directions:
Preheat oven to 350 F. In a bowl, mix almond and coconut flours and salt. Add in butter and mix until crumbly. Pour in the eggs one after another while mixing until formed into a ball. Flatten the dough on a clean flat surface, cover with plastic wrap, and refrigerate for 1 hour. Dust a clean flat surface with almond flour, unwrap the dough and roll out into a large rectangle. Fit into a greased pie pan and with a fork, prick the base of the crust. Bake for 15 minutes; let cool. For the filling, melt butter in a skillet over medium-low heat and sauté onion and garlic for 3 minutes. Add in mushrooms, bell pepper, and green beans; cook for 5 minutes. In a bowl, beat heavy cream, sour cream, almond milk, and eggs. Season with salt, pepper, and nutmeg. Stir in parsley and Monterey Jack cheese. Spread the mushroom mixture on the baked pastry and spread the cheese filling on top. Place the pie in the oven and bake for 35 minutes. Slice and serve.
Per serving: Cal 531; Net Carbs 6.5g; Fat 39g; Protein 21g

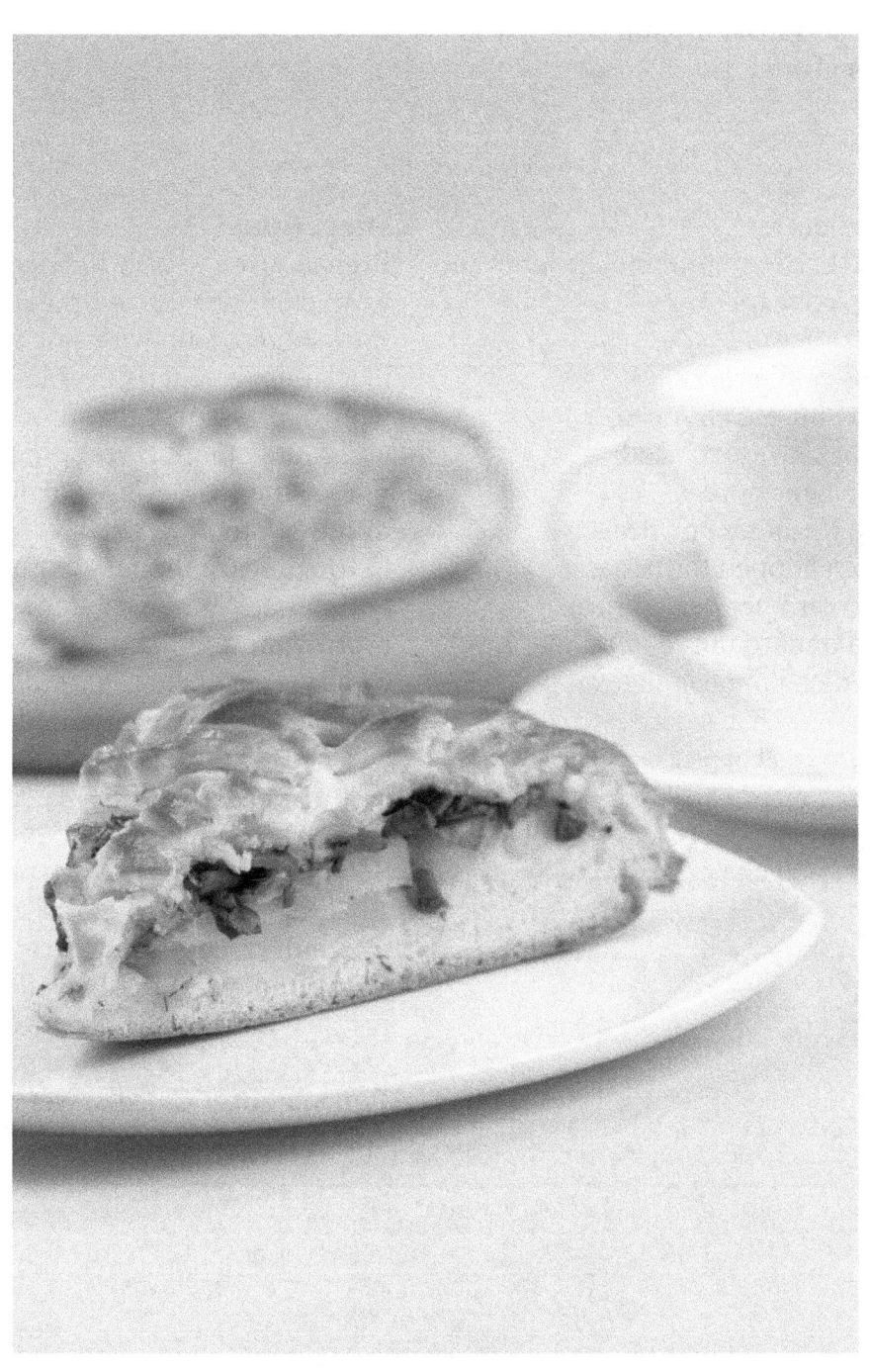

Vegetable Biryani

Prep. Time: 75 min
Servings: 4

Ingredients:
1 cup sliced cremini mushrooms
2 tbsp olive oil
3 tbsp ghee
6 cups cauli rice
1 white onion, chopped
2 garlic cloves, minced
1 tsp ginger puree
1 tbsp turmeric powder
2 cups chopped tomatoes
1 habanero pepper, minced
1 tbsp tomato puree
1 cup diced paneer cheese
½ cup spinach, chopped
½ cup kale, chopped
¼ cup chopped parsley
1 cup Greek yogurt
Salt and black pepper to taste

Directions:
Preheat oven to 400 F. Microwave cauli rice for 1 minute. Remove and season with salt and black pepper; set aside. Melt ghee in a pan over medium heat and sauté onion, garlic, ginger puree, and turmeric. Cook for 5 minutes, stirring regularly. Add in tomatoes, habanero pepper, and tomato puree; cook for 5 more minutes. Stir in mushrooms, paneer cheese, spinach, kale, and 1/3 cup water and simmer for 15 minutes or until the mushrooms soften. Turn the heat off and stir in yogurt. Spoon half of the mixture into a baking dish. Spread half of the cauli rice on top. Repeat the layers and top with olive oil and parsley. Bake for 25 minutes. Serve.
Per serving: Cal 351; Net Carbs 2g; Fat 19g; Protein 16g

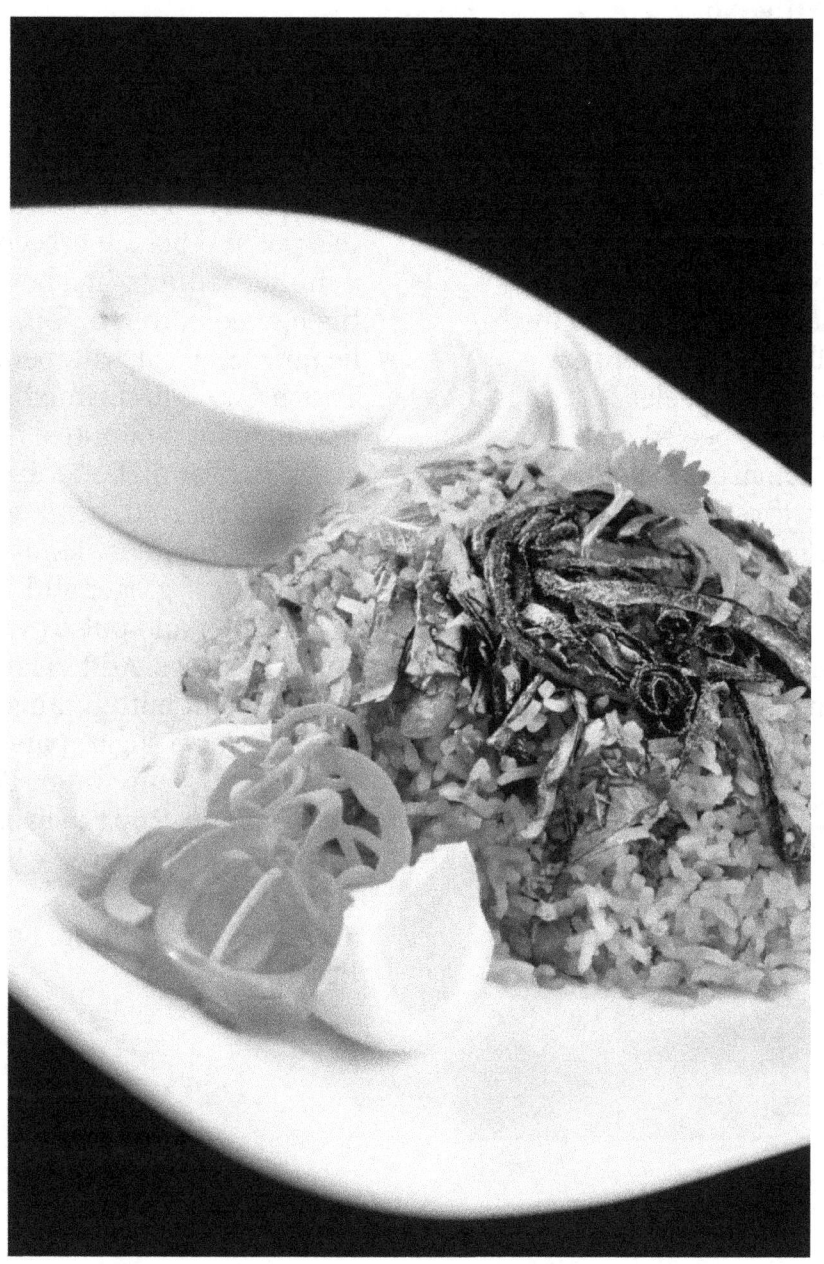

Charred Broccoli with Tamarind Sauce

Prep. Time: 30 min
Servings: 6

Ingredients:
1 head broccoli, cut into "steaks"
4 tbsp melted butter
½ cup peanut butter
1 white onion, finely chopped
1 small red chili, chopped
1 garlic clove, peeled
inch ginger, peeled
2 tbsp tamarind sauce
1 tsp Swerve brown sugar
1 tsp garlic powder
1 tsp dried basil
3 tbsp parsley, chopped
½ lemon, juiced
Salt and black pepper to taste

Directions:
Bring to a boil 2 cups of water in a pot and blanch broccoli for 2 minutes; drain. In a bowl, mix the melted butter, onion, garlic powder, basil, salt, pepper. Toss broccoli in the mixture and marinate for 5 minutes. Heat a grill pan over high. Cook broccoli until charred, turning once, about 6-8 minutes. Transfer to a plate. Place ginger and garlic in a blender and pulse until broken into pieces. Add in lemon juice, peanut butter, tamarind sauce, Swerve sugar, parsley, chili, and 1/3 cup water. Blend until smooth. Top the broccoli with the sauce. Serve.

Per serving:
Cal 271; Net Carbs 5g; Fat 18g; Protein 7.6g

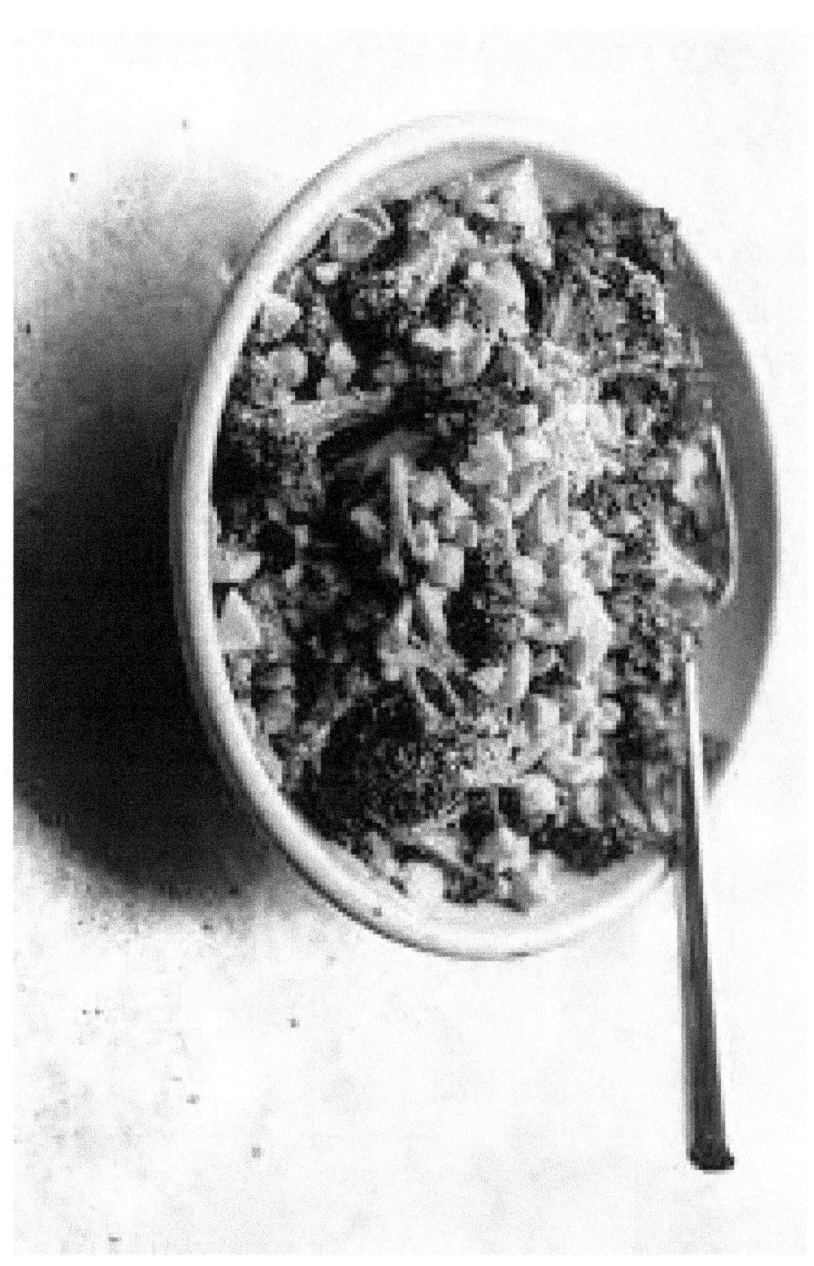

Chapter 4 Poultry & Meat

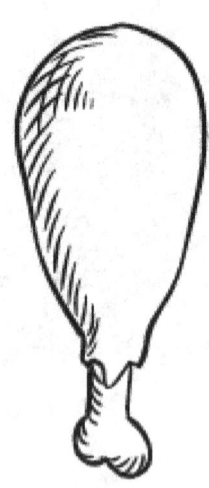

Citrus Pork with Cabbage & Tomatoes

Prep.Time: 25 minutes
Servings: 2

Ingredients:
3 tbsp olive oil
2 tbsp lemon juice
1 garlic clove, pureed
2 pork loin chops
1/3 head cabbage, shredded
1 tomato, chopped
1 tbsp white wine
Salt and black pepper to taste
¼ tsp cumin
¼ tsp ground nutmeg
1 tbsp parsley

Directions:
In a large bowl, mix the lemon juice, garlic, salt, pepper, and 1 tbsp of olive oil. Brush the pork with the mixture. Preheat grill to high heat. Grill the pork for 2 minutes on each side until cooked through. Remove to serving plates. Warm the remaining olive oil in a pan and cook the cabbage for 5 minutes. Drizzle with white wine, sprinkle with cumin, nutmeg, salt, and pepper. Add in the tomato and cook for 5-6 minutes, stirring occasionally. Place on a serving dish the sautéed cabbage to the side of the chops and serve sprinkled with parsley.

Per serving:
Cal 565; Fat 37g; Net Carbs 6.1g; Protein 43g

Baked Pork Sausage with Vegetables

Prep.Time: 45 minutes
Servings: 2

Ingredients:
1 tbsp olive oil
½ lb pork sausages
2 tomatoes, chopped
1 small onion, sliced
½ medium carrot, sliced
1 tsp smoked paprika
1 red bell peppers, sliced
1 sprig rosemary, chopped
1 garlic clove, minced
1 tbsp balsamic vinegar
Salt and black pepper to taste

Directions:
Preheat the oven to 360 F. Heat olive oil in a saucepan and add the tomatoes, bell peppers, garlic, carrot, onion, and balsamic vinegar, and cook for 8-10 minutes until softened and lightly golden. Season with salt, paprika, and pepper. Transfer to a baking dish. Arrange the sausages on top of the veggies. Place the dish in the oven and cook for 20-25 minutes until the sausages have browned to the desired color. Serve topped with rosemary.

Per serving:
Cal 411; Fat 32g; Net Carbs 6.5g; Protein 15g

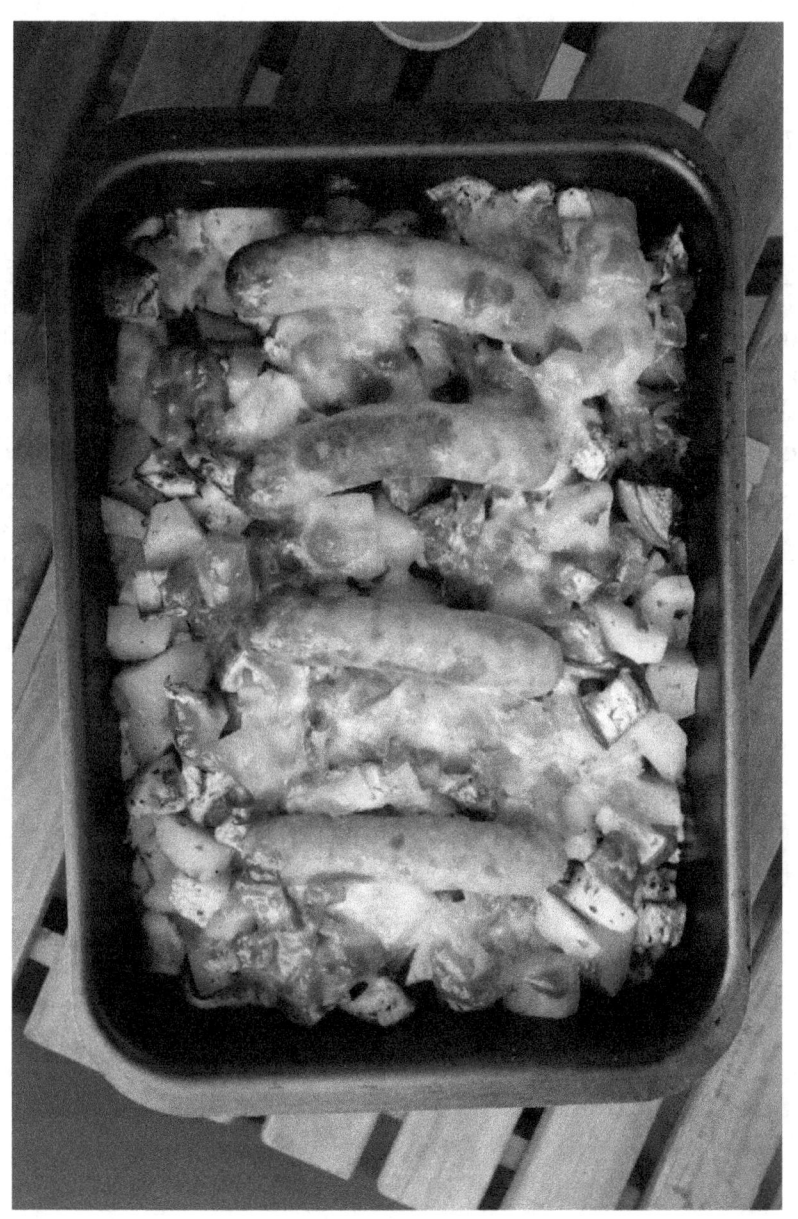

Pork Chops with Basil-Tomato Sauce

Prep.Time: 45 minutes
Servings: 2

Ingredients:
2 pork chops
½ tbsp fresh basil, chopped
1 garlic clove, minced
1 tbsp olive oil
7 oz canned diced tomatoes
½ tbsp tomato paste
Salt and black pepper to taste
½ red chili, finely chopped

Directions:
Season the pork with pepper and salt. Set a pan over medium-low heat and warm oil. Place in the pork chops and cook for 3-4 minutes. Turn and bake for another 3-4 minutes; remove to a bowl. Cook for 30 seconds after adding garlic to pan. Stir in the tomato paste, tomatoes, and chili. Bring to a boil and reduce the heat. Place in the pork chops, cover the pan, and simmer everything for 30 minutes. Remove the pork chops to plates and sprinkle with fresh basil to serve.

Per serving:
Cal 425; Fat 25g; Net Carbs 2.5g; Protein 39g

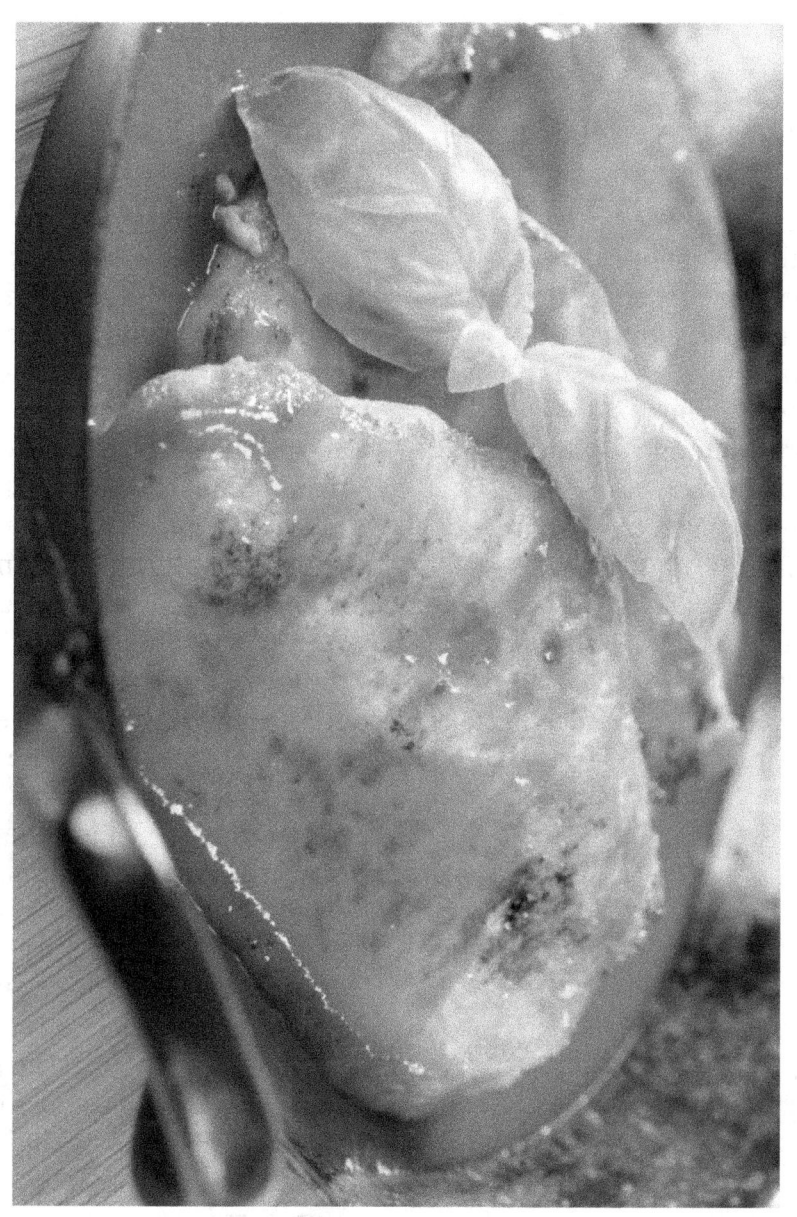

Herb Pork Chops with Cranberry Sauce

Prep.Time: 2 hours and 45 minutes
Servings: 2

Ingredients:
2 pork chops
½ tsp garlic powder
Salt and black pepper to taste
1 tsp fresh basil, chopped
A drizzle of olive oil
½ onion, chopped
½ cup white wine
Juice of ½ lemon
1 bay leaf
1 cup chicken stock
1 tbsp parsley, chopped
1 cup cranberries
1 tsp fresh rosemary, chopped
½ cup xylitol
½ cup water
½ tsp sriracha sauce

Directions:
Preheat oven to 340 F. In a bowl, combine the pork with basil, salt, garlic powder, and black pepper. Place a drizzle of oil to a pan and heat it over medium heat, place in the pork, and cook until browned, about 4-5 minutes; set aside. Cook the onion in the pan for 2 minutes. Place in the bay leaf and wine and cook for 4 minutes. Pour in chicken stock and lemon juice and simmer for 5 minutes. Return the pork and cook for 10 minutes. Cover the pan and transfer it in the oven for 2 hours. Uncover and bake for 5 minutes. Set another pan over medium heat, add in the cranberries, rosemary, sriracha sauce, water, and xylitol and bring to a simmer for 15 minute. Remove the pork chops from the oven and discard the bay leaf. Pour the sauce over the pork and serve sprinkled with parsley.

Per serving:
Cal 450; Fat 24g; Net Carbs 7.3g; Protein 42g

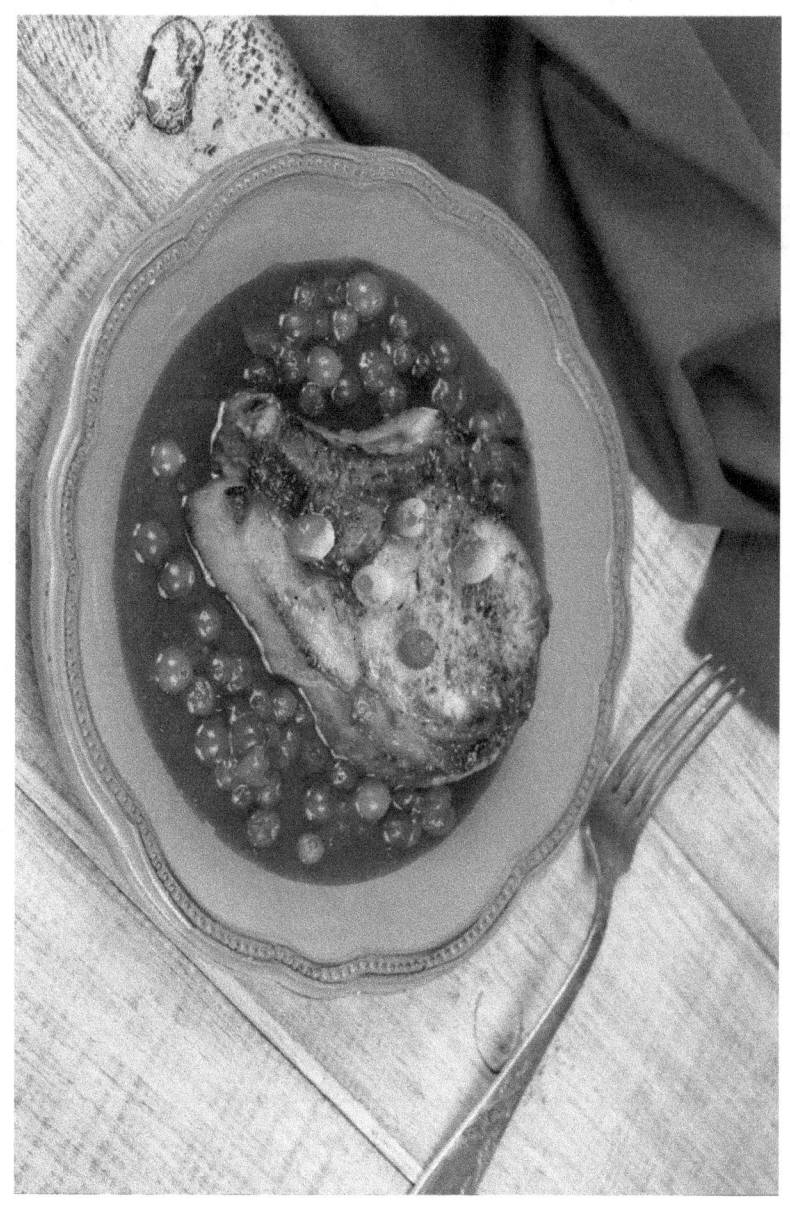

Barbecued Pork Chops

Prep.Time: 20 minutes
Servings: 2

Ingredients:
2 pork loin chops, boneless
½ cup BBQ sauce, sugar-free
Salt and black pepper to taste
½ tsp ginger powder
½ tsp onion powder
½ tsp garlic powder
1 tsp red pepper flakes
2 thyme sprigs, chopped

Directions:
Mix black pepper, salt, ginger powder, onion powder, garlic powder, and red pepper flakes in a small bowl. Rub the spices onto the pork chops. Preheat the grill to high. Place and cook the meat for 2 minutes per side. Reduce the heat to medium and brush the BBQ sauce on the meat, cover, and grill for another 5 minutes. Open the lid, turn the meatp and brush again with barbecue sauce. Continue cooking covered for 5 minutes. Remove and serve sprinkled with thyme.

Per serving:
Cal 412; Fat 35g; Net Carbs 1.1g; Protein 34g

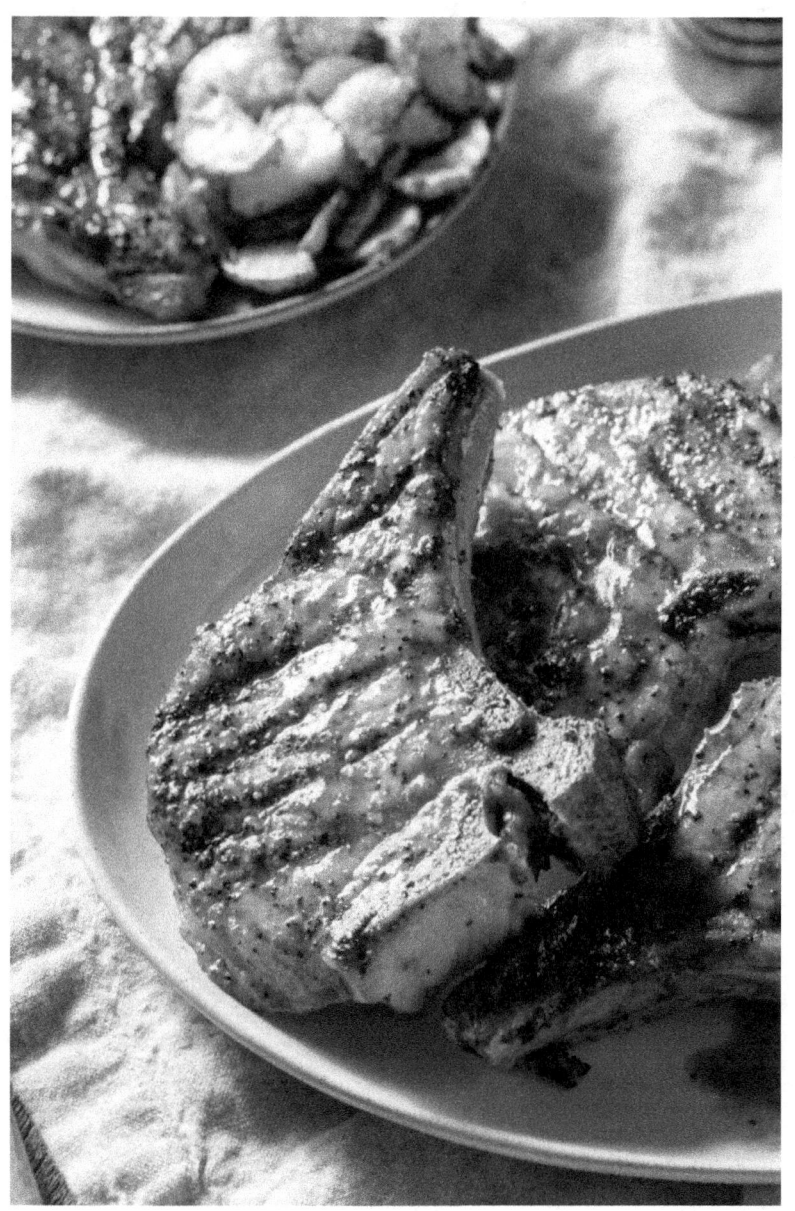

Chapter 5 Fish & Seafood

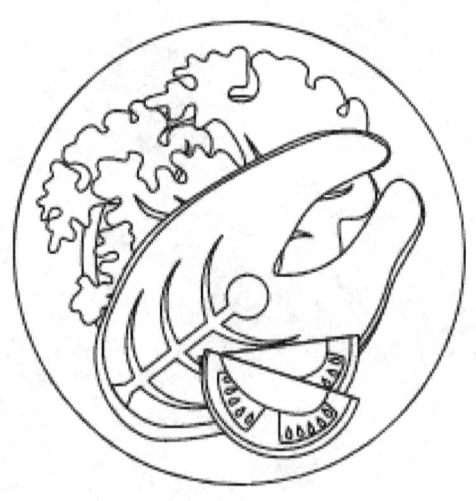

Parmesan Shrimp Scampi Pizza

Prep. Time: 30 min
Servings: 4

Ingredients:
3 tbsp olive oil
2 tbsp butter
½ lb shrimp, deveined
½ cup almond flour
¼ tsp salt
2 tbsp ground psyllium husk
2 garlic cloves, minced
¼ cup white wine
½ tsp dried basil
½ tsp dried parsley
½ lemon, juiced
2 cups grated cheese blend
½ tsp Italian seasoning
¼ cup grated Parmesan

Instructions:
Preheat oven to 370/380 F. Line a baking sheet with parchment paper. In a bowl, mix almond flour, salt, psyllium powder, 1 tbsp of olive oil, and 1 cup of lukewarm water until dough forms. Spread the mixture on the baking sheet and bake for 10 minutes. Meanwhile, heat butter and the remaining olive oil in a skillet. Sauté garlic for 30 seconds. Mix in the wine and cook until it reduces by half. Stir in basil, parsley, and lemon juice. Stir in the shrimp and cook for 3 minutes. Mix in the cheese blend and Italian seasoning. Let the cheese melt, 3 minutes. Spread the shrimp mixture on the crust and top with Parmesan cheese. Bake for 5 minutes or until the cheese melts. Slice and serve warm.

Per serving:
Cal 419; Net Carbs 3g; Fats 29g; Protein 23g

Quick Tuna Omelet

Prep. Time: 20 min
Servings: 2

Ingredients:
1 avocado, sliced
1 tbsp chopped chives
1/3 cup canned tuna, drained
¼ tsp smoked cayenne pepper
4 eggs, beaten
4 tbsp mascarpone cheese
1 tbsp butter
Salt and black pepper, to taste

Instructions:
Cook the butter in a pan over medium heat. Pour in the eggs and cook for 3 minutes. Flip the omelet and continue to cook for 2 more minutes or until golden. Sprinkle with cayenne pepper, salt and pepper. Slide the omelet onto a plate and spread the mascarpone cheese over. Top with tuna, avocado, and chives. To cover the filling, fold the omelet in half and serve.

Per serving:
Cal 481; Fat 38g; Net Carbs 6.2g; Protein 279g

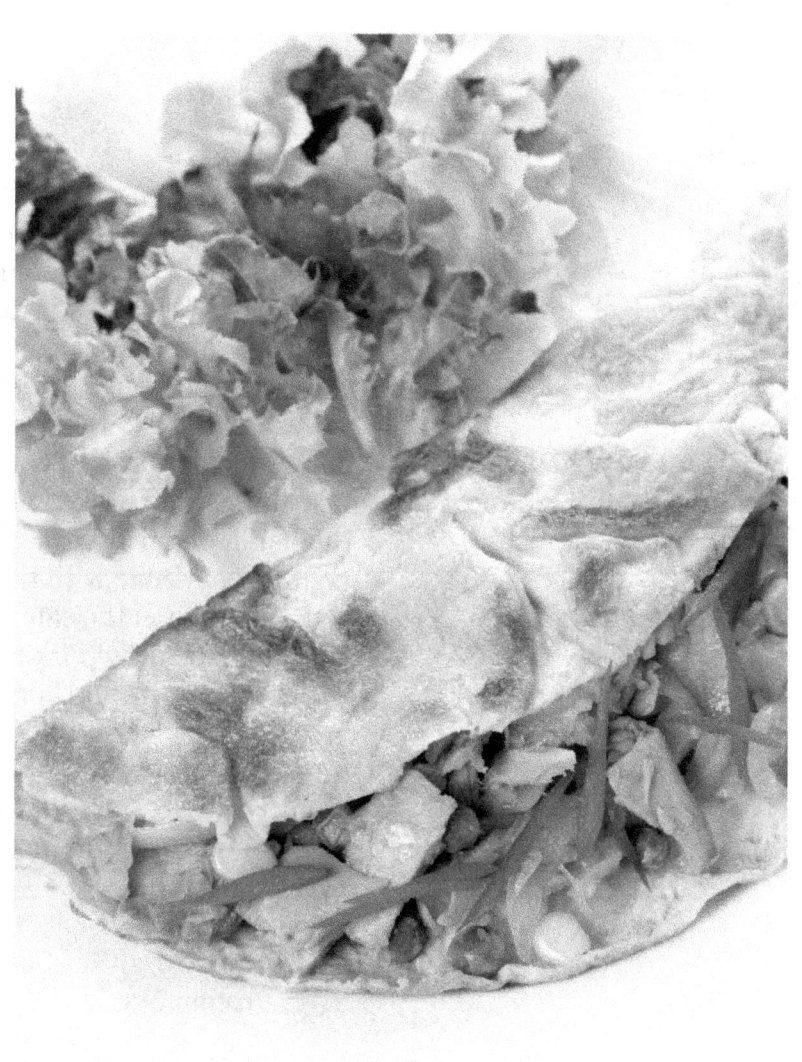

Baked Haddock with Cheesy Topping

Prep. Time: 35 min
Servings: 4

Ingredients:
1 tbsp butter
1 shallot, sliced
1 lb haddock fillets
2 eggs, hard-boiled, chopped
3 tbsp hazelnut flour
2 cups sour cream
1 tbsp parsley, chopped
½ cup pork rinds, crushed
1 cup mozzarella cheese, grated
Salt and black pepper to taste

Directions:
Cook butter in a saucepan over medium-low heat and sauté the shallot for 3 minutes. Reduce the heat to low and stir in the hazelnut flour to form a roux. Cook the roux until golden brown and stir in the sour cream until smooth. Season to taste, and add parsley. Arrange the haddock on a greased baking dish, sprinkle with the eggs, and spoon the sauce over. In a bowl, mix the pork rinds with mozzarella, and spread the mixture over the sauce. Bake in the oven for 20 minutes at 370 F until the top is golden and the sauce and cheese are bubbly. Serve warm.

Per serving:
Cal 788; Fat 57g; Net Carbs 8.5g; Protein 65g

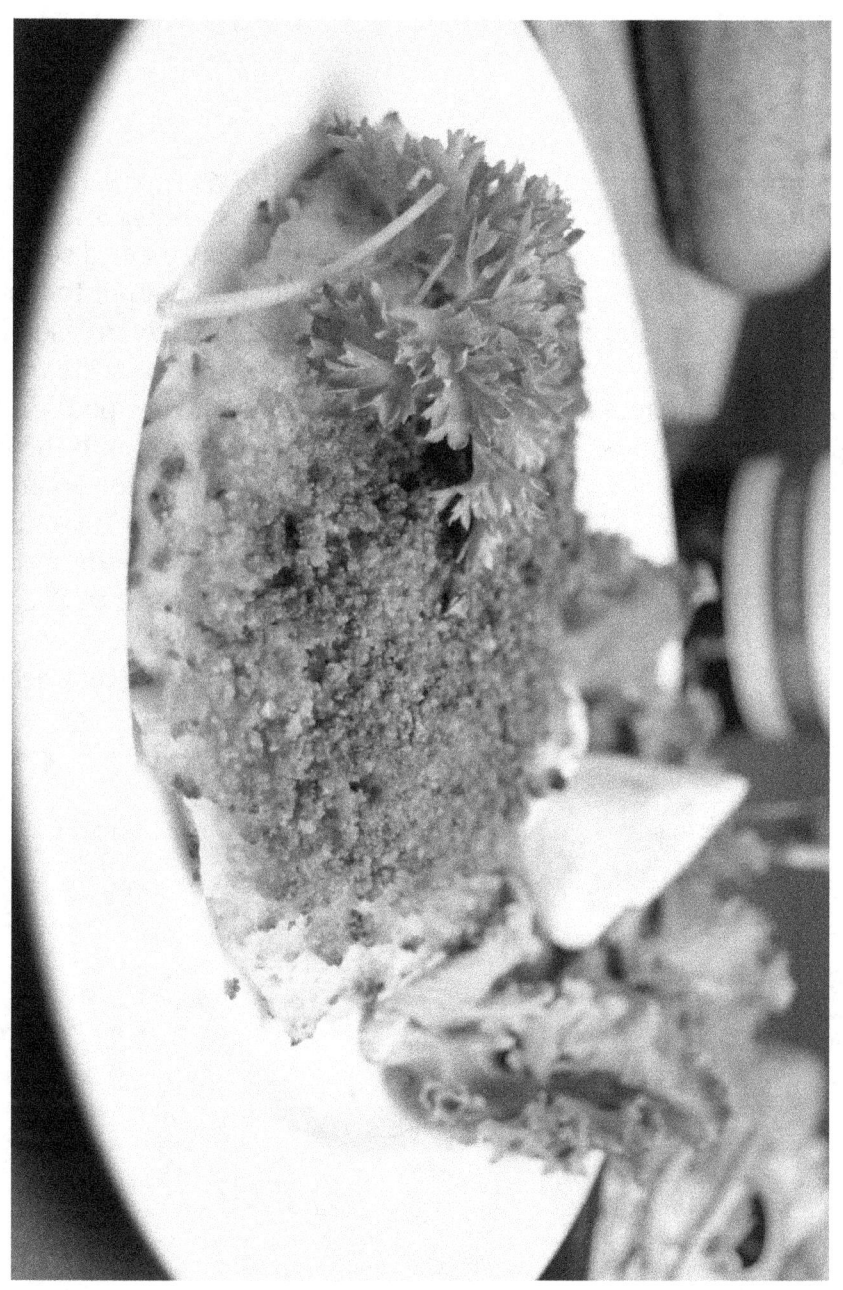

Baked Cod with Parmesan and Almonds

Prep. Time: 40 min
Servings: 2

Ingredients:
2 cod fillets
1 cup Brussels sprouts
1 tbsp butter, melted
Salt and black pepper to taste
1 cup heavy cream
2 tbsp Parmesan cheese, grated
2 tbsp shaved almonds

Directions:
Toss the fish fillets and Brussels sprouts in butter and season with salt and pepper to taste. Spread them on a greased baking dish. Mix heavy cream with Parmesan cheese; pour and smear the cream onto the fish. Bake in the oven for 20/25 minutes at 400 F. Take the dish out, sprinkle with almonds, and bake for 3-5 minutes. Serve.

Per serving:
Cal 560; Fat 45g; Net Carbs 5.4g; Protein 25g

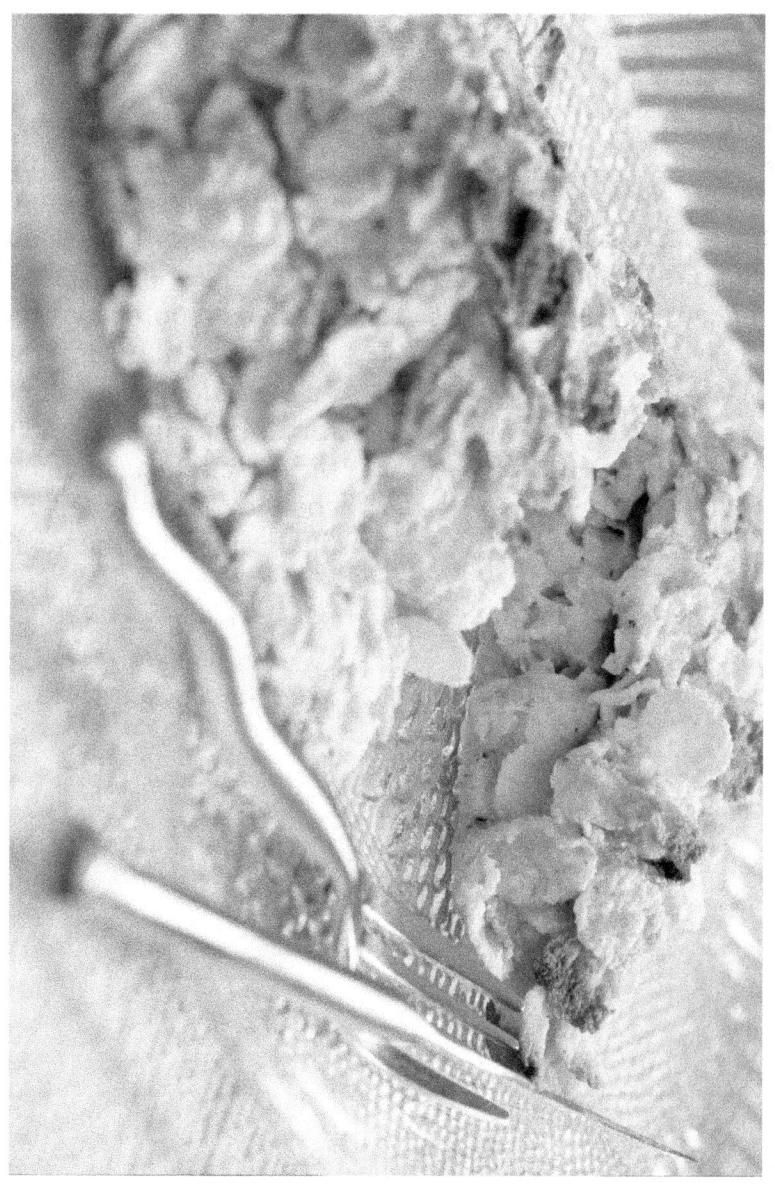

Greek Sea Bass with Olive Sauce

Prep. Time: 20 min
Servings: 2

Ingredients:
2 sea bass fillets
2 tbsp olive oil
A pinch of chili pepper
1 tbsp green olives, sliced
1 lemon, juiced
Salt to taste

Directions:
Preheat grill to high. In a bowl, mix together chili pepper, half of the olive oil, salt and rub onto the sea bass fillets. Grill the fish on both sides for 5-6 minutes until brown. In a skillet over medium heat, warm the remaining olive oil and stir in the lemon juice, olives, and salt; cook for 3-4 minutes. Plate the fillets and pour the lemon sauce over to serve.

Per serving:
Cal 267; Fat 16g; Net Carbs 1.6g; Protein 24g

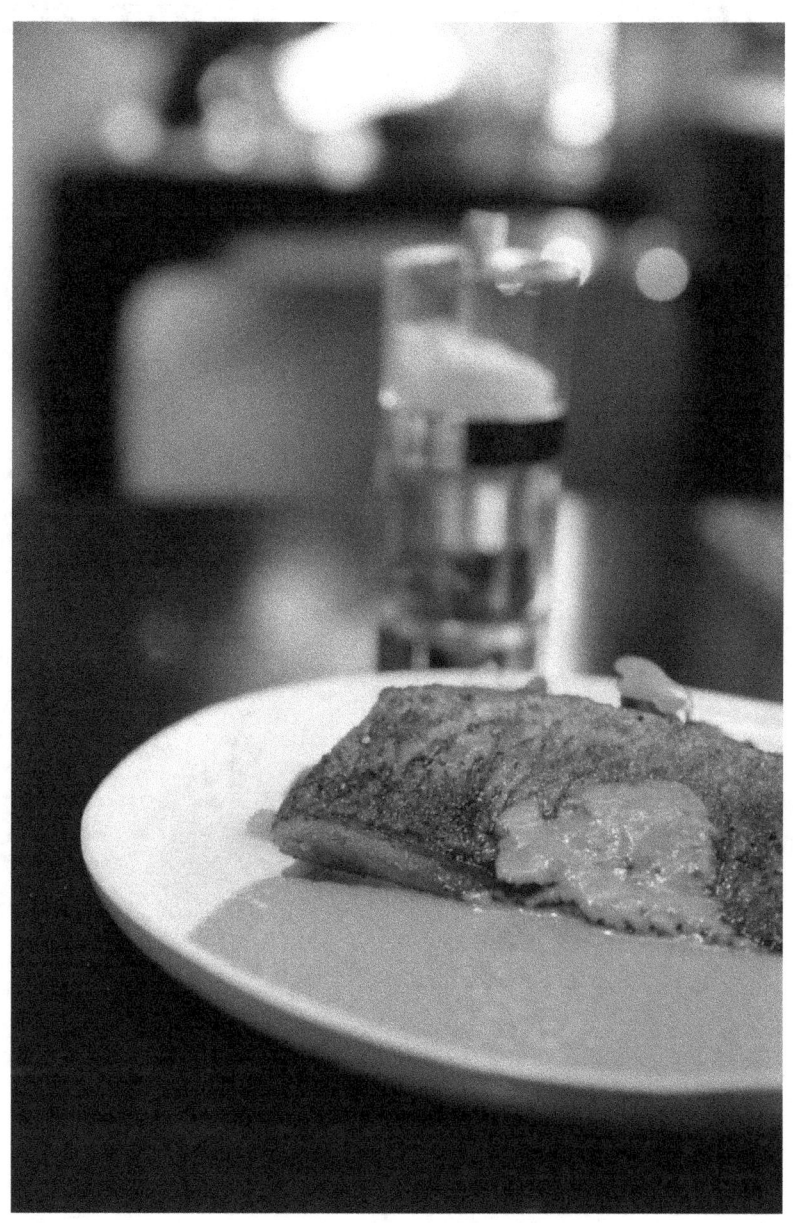

Chapter 6 Snacks, Appetizers & Side Dishes

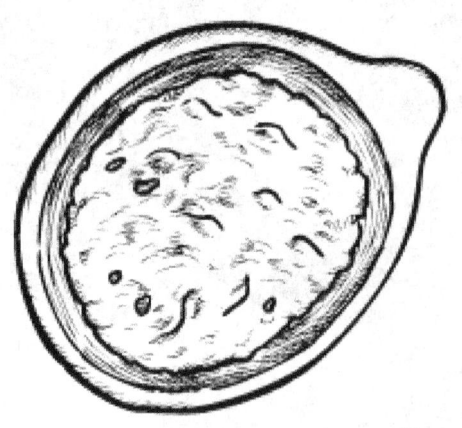

Maple Tahini Straws

Prep.Time: 30 minutes
Servings: 4

Ingredients:
For the puff pastry
3 tbsp coconut flour
¼ cup almond flour
½ tsp xanthan gum
3 whole eggs
4 tbsp cream cheese, softened
¼ teaspoon cream of tartar
¼ cup butter, cold
3 tbsp erythritol
1 tsp vanilla extract
½ tsp salt
For the filling
2 tbsp sugar-free maple syrup
2 tbsp poppy seeds
2 tbsp sesame seeds
1 egg, beaten
3 tbsp tahini

Directions:
Preheat oven to 345/350 F. Line a baking tray with parchment paper. In a bowl, mix almond and coconut flours, xanthan gum, and salt. Add in cream cheese, cream of tartar, and butter; mix with an electric mixer until crumbly. Add erythritol and vanilla extract until mixed. Then, pour in 3 eggs one after another while mixing until formed into a ball. Flatten the dough on a clean flat surface, cover with plastic wrap, and refrigerate for 1 hour. Dust a clean flat surface with almond flour, unwrap the dough, and roll out the dough into a large rectangle. In a bowl, mix maple syrup and tahini and spread the mixture over the pastry. Sprinkle with half of the sesame seeds and cut the dough into 16 strips. Fold each strip in half. Brush the top with the beaten egg, sprinkle with the remaining seeds and poppy seeds. Twist the pastry three to four times into straws and place on the baking sheet. Bake until golden brown, 15 minutes. Serve with chocolate sauce.

Per serving:
Cal 351; Net Carbs 3.1g, Fat 31g, Protein 11g

Basil Spinach & Zucchini Lasagna

Prep.Time: 50 minutes
Servings: 4

Ingredients:
2 zucchinis, sliced
Salt and black pepper to taste
2 cups feta cheese
2 cups mozzarella, shredded
3 cups tomato sauce
1 cup spinach
1 tbsp basil, chopped

Directions:
Preheat oven to 370 F. Mix feta, mozzarella cheese, salt, and pepper to evenly combine and spread ¼ cup of the mixture at the bottom of a greased baking dish. Layer 1/3 of the zucchini slices on top, spread 1 cup of tomato sauce over, and scatter a 1/3 cup of spinach on top. Repeat the layering process two more times to exhaust the ingredients while finally making sure to layer with the last ¼ cup of cheese mixture. Bake for 35 minutes until the cheese has a nice golden brown color. Remove the dish, sit for 5 minutes and serve sprinkled with basil.

Per serving:
Cal 411; Fat 43g; Net Carbs 3.2g; Protein 6.5g

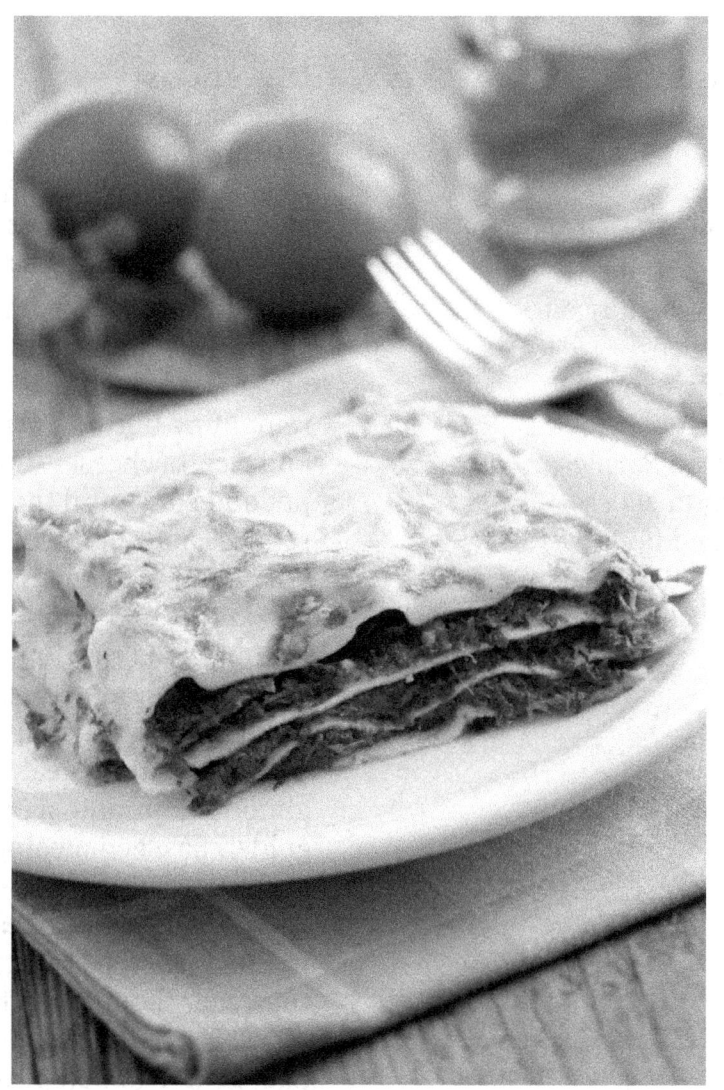

Cauli Rice Arancini

Prep.Time: 30 minutes
Servings: 4

Ingredients:
2 tbsp butter
2 tbsp olive oil
2 eggs
1 white onion, finely chopped
2 scallions, chopped
2 garlic cloves, minced
1 cup cauli rice
¼ cup white wine
¼ cup vegetable stock
¼ cup grated Parmesan
½ cup ricotta cheese
1 cup almond flour
½ cup golden flaxseed meal
Salt and black pepper to taste

Directions:
Heat butter in a saucepan over medium heat. Stir in garlic and onion and cook until fragrant and soft, 3 minutes. Mix in cauli rice for 30 seconds; add in wine, stir, allow reduction and absorption into cauli rice. Add in vegetable stock, salt, pepper, remaining butter, Parmesan and ricotta cheeses. Cover the pot and cook until the liquid reduces and the "rice" thickens. Open the lid, stir well, and spoon the mixture into a bowl to cool. Mold the dough into mini patties, 14-16 pieces; set aside. Heat olive oil in a skillet over medium heat. Pour the almond flour onto a plate, the golden flaxseed meal in another, and beat the eggs in a medium bowl. Lightly dredge each patty in the flour, then in eggs, and then coat them in the flaxseed meal. Fry in the oil until compacted and golden brown, 2 minutes per side. Garnish with scallions and serve.

Per serving:
Cal 359; Net Carbs 6.2g, Fat 29g, Protein 13g

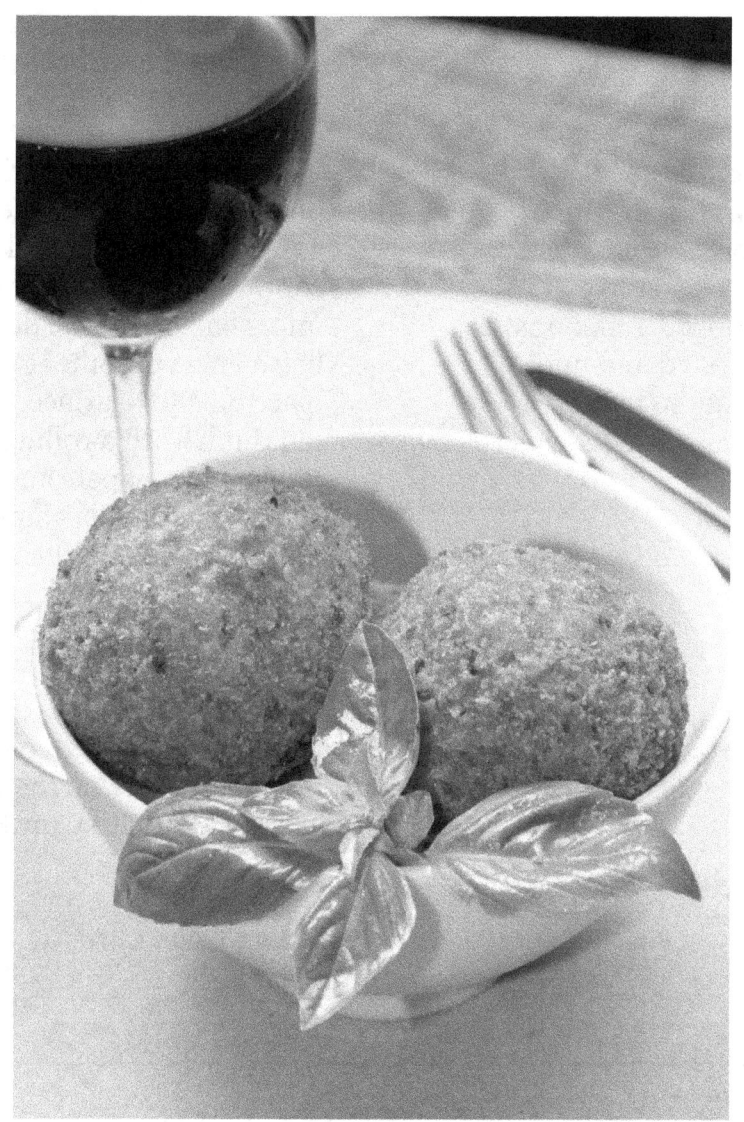

Flaxseed Toasts with Avocado Paté

Prep.Time: 25 minutes
Servings: 4

Ingredients:
1 pinch of salt
½ cup flaxseed meal
For the avocado paté
3 ripe avocados, chopped
4 tbsp Greek yogurt
2 tbsp chopped green onions
1 lemon, zested and juiced
Black pepper to taste
Smoked paprika to garnish

Directions:
Preheat oven to 350/360 F. Place a skillet over medium heat. Put in flaxseed meal, ¼ cup water, and salt and mix continually to form the dough into a ball. Place the dough between 2 parchment papers, place on a flat surface, and flatten thinly with a rolling pin. Remove the papers and cut the pastry into tortilla chips. Place on a baking sheet and bake for 8-12 minutes or until crispy. In a bowl, mix avocados, yogurt, green onions, lemon zest and juice, and black pepper until evenly combined. Spread the paté on the toasts and garnish with paprika. Serve immediately.

Per serving:
Cal 359; Net Carbs 4g, Fat 31g, Protein 7g

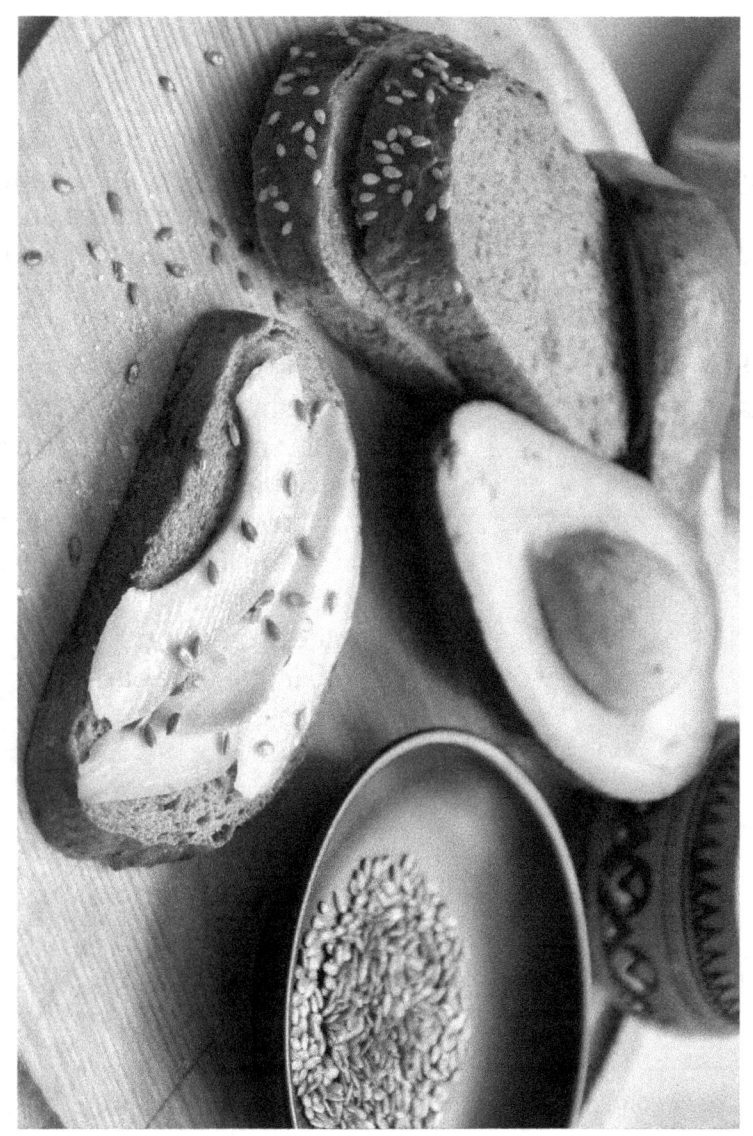

Caramelized Onion & Cream Cheese Spread

Prep.Time: 35 minutes
Servings: 4

Ingredients:
2 cups sour cream
8 oz cream cheese, softened
½ tbsp Worcestershire sauce
2 tbsp butter
3 yellow onions, thinly sliced
1 tsp Swerve sugar
¼ cup white wine
Salt to taste

Directions:
Melt the butter in a skillet over medium heat. Add in the onions, Swerve sugar, and salt. Cook with frequent stirring for 10-15 minutes. Add in white wine, stir, and allow sizzling out, 10 minutes. In a serving bowl, mix sour cream and cream cheese. Add in caramelized onions and Worcestershire sauce and stir well into the cream. Serve with celery sticks if desired.

Per serving:
Cal 379; Net Carbs 8g; Fat 34g; Protein 8g

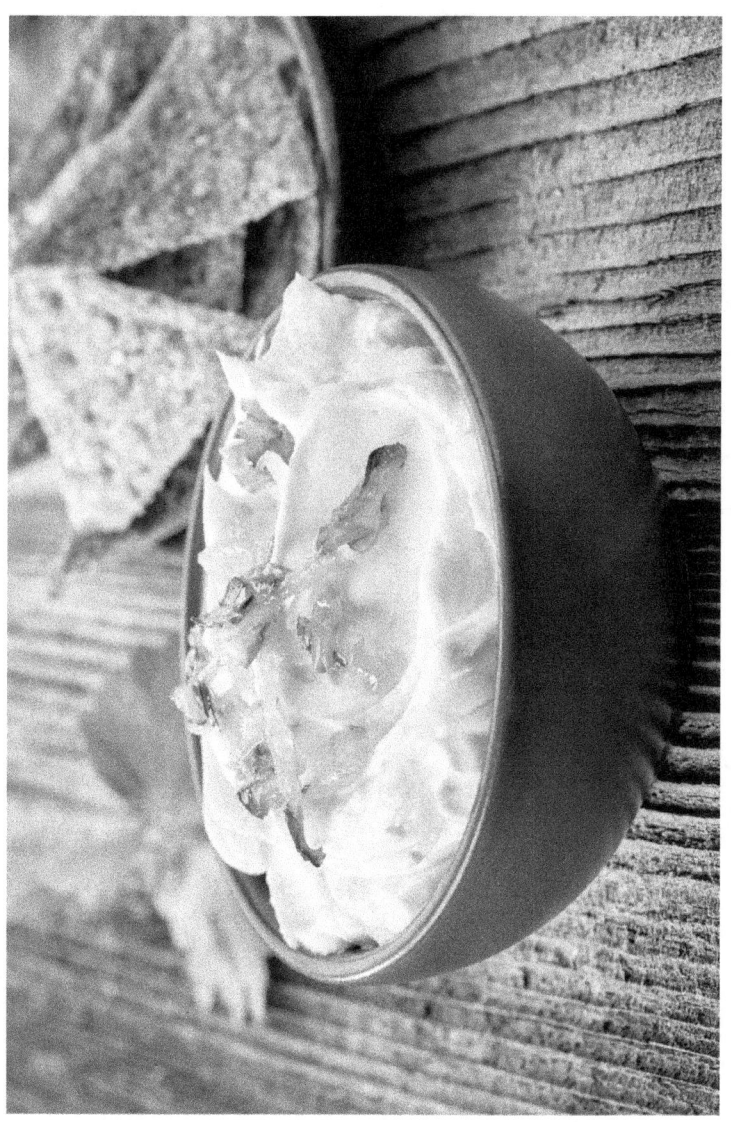

Chapter 7 Desserts, Fruits & Drinks

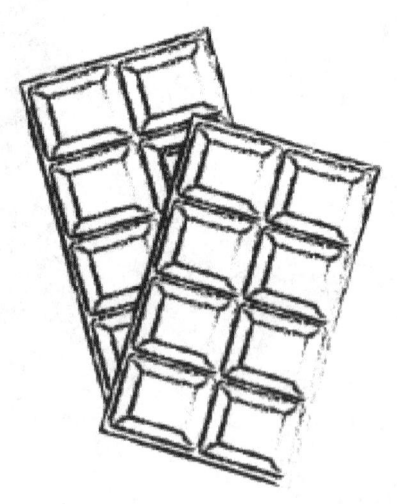

Chocolate Mousse Pots with Blackberries

Prep. Time: 20 min
Servings: 4

Ingredients:
2 ½ cups unsweetened dark chocolate, melted
½ cup Swerve confectioner's sugar
3 cups heavy cream
½ tsp vanilla extract
½ cup blackberries, chopped
Some blackberries for topping

Directions:
In a stand mixer, beat heavy cream and Swerve sugar until creamy. Add dark chocolate and vanilla extract and mix until smoothly combined. Fold in blackberries. Divide the mixture between 4 dessert cups, cover with plastic wrap, and refrigerate for 2 hours. Garnish with the reserved blackberries and serve.

Per serving:
Cal 309; Net Carbs 2.6g; Fat 33g; Protein 2g

Dark Chocolate Brownies

Prep. Time: 45 min
Servings: 4

Ingredients:
10 tbsp butter
2 oz sugar-free dark chocolate
2 eggs, beaten
¼ cup cocoa powder
½ cup almond flour
½ tsp baking powder
½ cup erythritol
½ tsp vanilla extract

Directions:
Preheat oven to 380 F. Line a baking sheet with parchment paper. In a bowl, mix cocoa powder, almond flour, baking powder, and erythritol until no lumps from the erythritol remain. In another bowl, add butter and dark chocolate and microwave for 30 seconds. Mix the eggs and vanilla into the chocolate mixture, then pour the mixture into the dry ingredients; mix well. Pour the batter onto the paper-lined sheet and bake for 20 minutes. Let cool completely and refrigerate for 2 hours. Slice into squares.

Per serving:
Cal 231; Net Carbs 3g; Fat 20g; Protein 4g

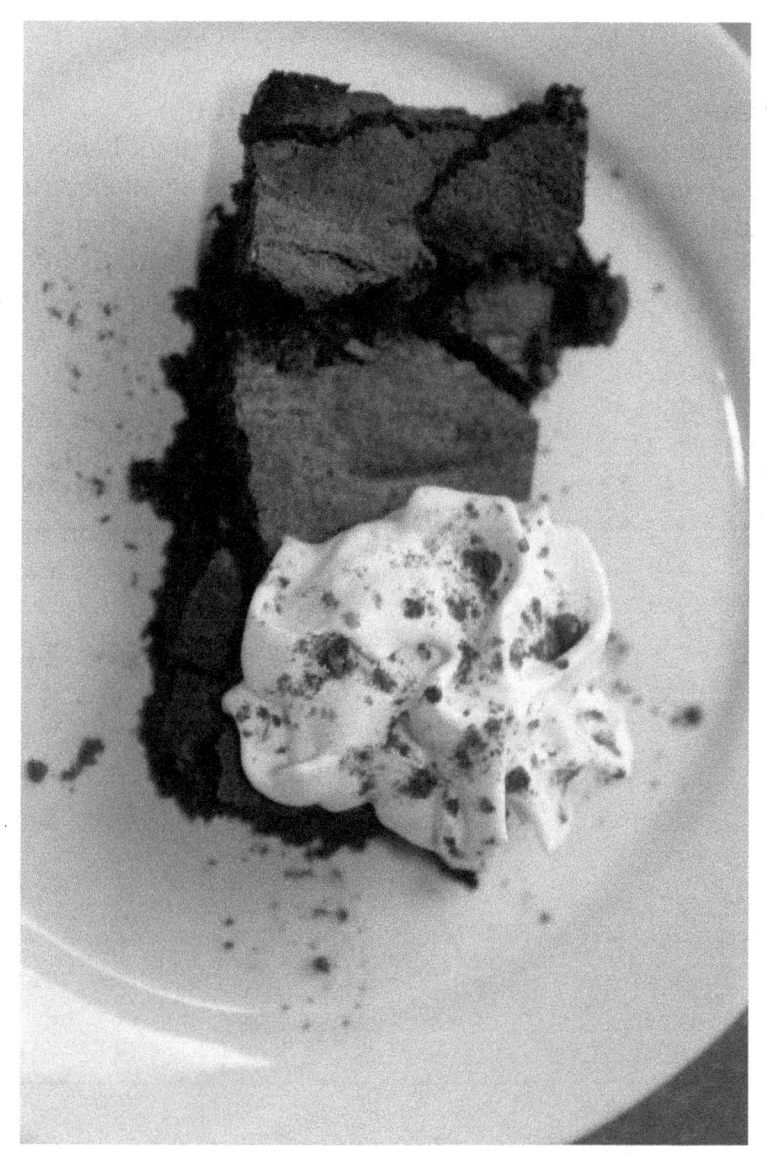

Favorite Peanut Butter Mousse

Prep. Time: 20 min
Servings: 4

Ingredients:
¼ cup smooth peanut butter
4 oz softened cream cheese
½ cup heavy cream
¼ cup xylitol
½ tsp vanilla extract

Directions:
Whip ½ cup of heavy cream in a bowl using an electric mixer until stiff peaks hole; set aside. In another bowl, beat cream cheese and peanut butter until creamy and smooth. Mix in xylitol and vanilla extract. Gradually fold in the cream mixture until well combined. If too thick, fold in 2 tbsp of the reserved heavy cream. Spoon the mousse into dessert glasses and serve.

Per serving:
Cal 229; Net Carbs 5g; Fat 21g; Protein 6g

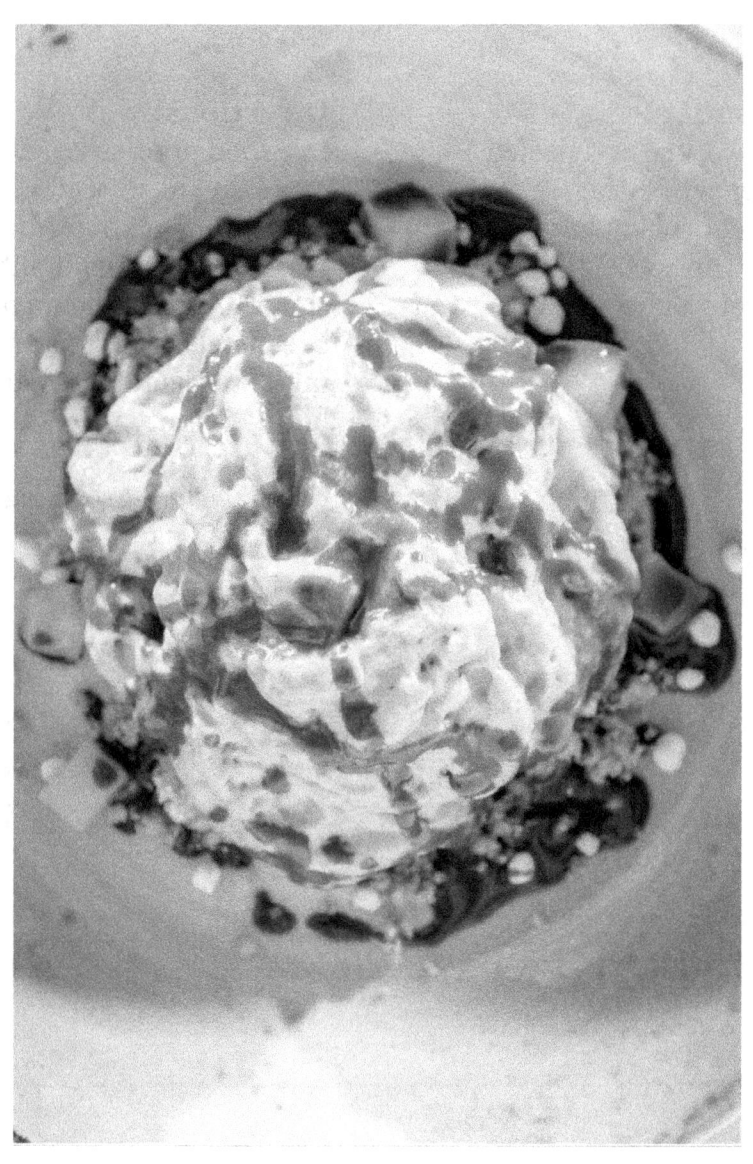

Avocado Mousse with Chocolate

Prep. Time: 20 min
Servings: 4

Ingredients:
1 avocado, pitted and peeled
2 tbsp cream of tartar
1 cup full-fat coconut cream
1 heaped tbsp cocoa powder
1 cup Greek yogurt

Directions:
In a food processor, add coconut cream, avocado, cocoa powder, cream of tartar, and Greek yogurt. Blend until smooth. Divide the mixture between 4 dessert cups and chill in the refrigerator for at least 2 hours. Serve.

Per serving:
Cal 329; Net Carbs 8.2g; Fat 31g; Protein 6g

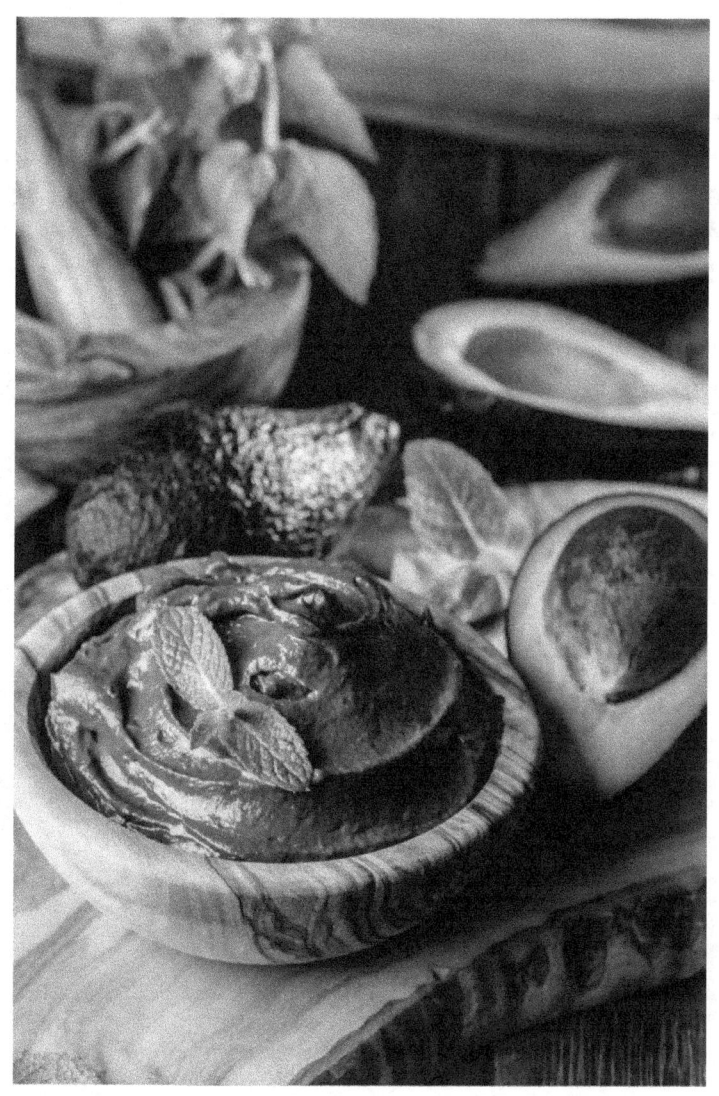

Mascarpone Cream Mousse

Prep. Time: 20 min
Servings: 6

Ingredients:
For the mascarpone
8 oz heavy cream
8 oz mascarpone cheese
4 tbsp cocoa powder
4 tbsp xylitol
For the vanilla mousse
3.5 oz heavy cream
3.5 oz cream cheese
1 tsp vanilla extract
2 tbsp xylitol

Directions:
Beat mascarpone cheese, heavy cream, cocoa powder, and xylitol with an electric mixer until creamy. Do not over mix, however. In another bowl, whisk all the mousse ingredients until smooth. Gradually fold vanilla mousse mixture into the mascarpone one until well incorporated. Spoon into dessert cups and serve.

Per serving:
Cal 409; Net Carbs 5.9g; Fat 32g; Protein 7.9g

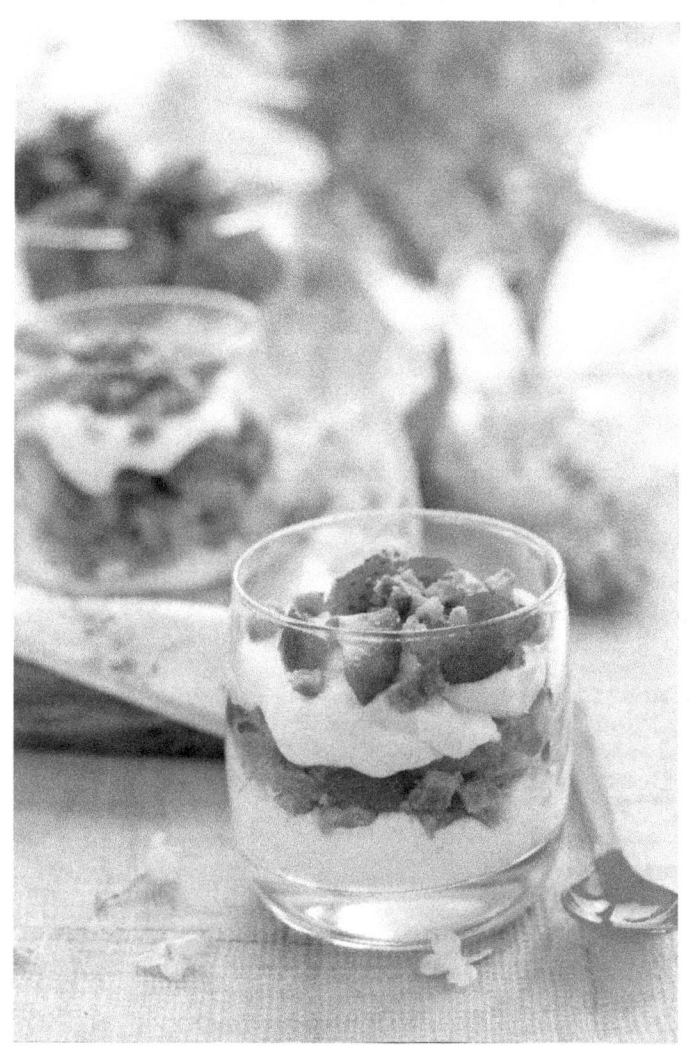

Chapter 8 Lunch

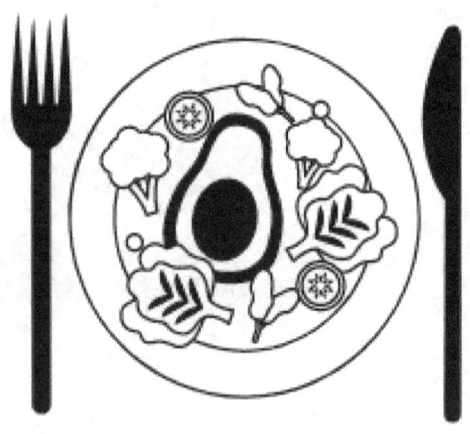

Marinara Turkey Linguine

Prep.Time: 20 minutes
Servings: 4

Ingredients:
½ cup Pecorino Romano cheese, grated
1 tsp olive oil
1 lb ground turkey
¾ tsp kosher salt
¼ onion, diced
1 clove garlic, minced
t cups marinara sauce
16 oz linguine, halved

Directions:
Warm the olive oil in your Instant Pot on Sauté. Brown the ground turkey until no longer pink or about 3 minutes. Stir in garlic and onion and cook for 4 minutes. Pour linguine, marinara sauce, salt, and 4 cups of water and seal the lid. Select Manual and cook for 5 minutes on High. Once done, perform a quick pressure release and unlock the lid. Serve topped with Pecorino Romano.

Pasta Tortiglioni with Beef & Black Beans

Prep.Time: 25 minutes
Servings: 4

Ingredients:
2 tbsp olive oil
1 lb ground beef
16 oz tortiglioni pasta
15 oz tomato sauce
15-oz canned black beans
15-oz canned corn, drained
10 oz red enchilada sauce
4 oz diced green chiles
1 cup shredded mozzarella
Salt and pepper to taste
2 tbsp Parmesan, grated
2 tbsp chopped parsley

Directions:
Heat oil on Sauté. Add ground beef and cook for 7 minutes. Mix in pasta, tomato sauce, enchilada sauce, black beans, 2 cups water, corn, and green chiles and stir. Seal the lid and cook on High Pressure for 10 minutes. Do a quick pressure release. Mix in mozzarella until melted and add pepper and salt. Garnish with parsley and Parmesan cheese.

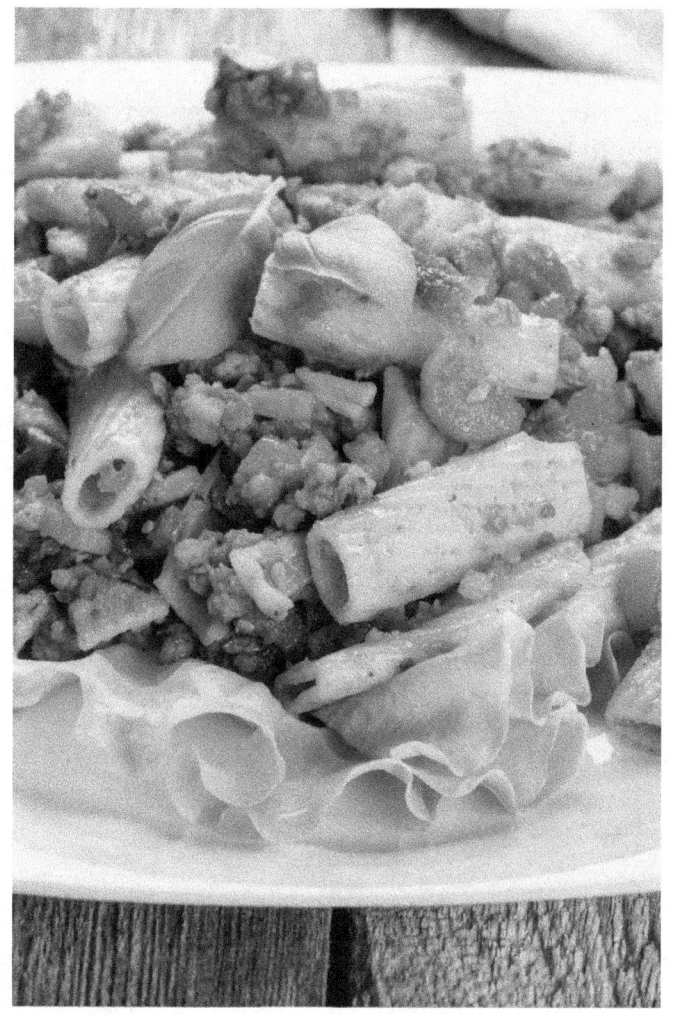

Mustard Macaroni & Cheese

Prep.Time: 20 minutes
Servings: 4

Ingredients:
16 oz elbow macaroni
1 cup heavy cream
Salt and pepper to taste
1 tbsp butter
1 tsp mustard powder
3 cups cheddar, shredded
½ cup Parmesan, grated

Directions:
Place macaroni and 4 cups of water in your Instant Pot. Sprinkle with salt and pepper and seal the lid. Select Manual and cook for 4 minutes on High. Once done, perform a quick pressure release. Mix in heavy cream, butter, mustard powder, and cheddar and let sit for 5 minutes. Sprinkle with Parmesan cheese and serve.

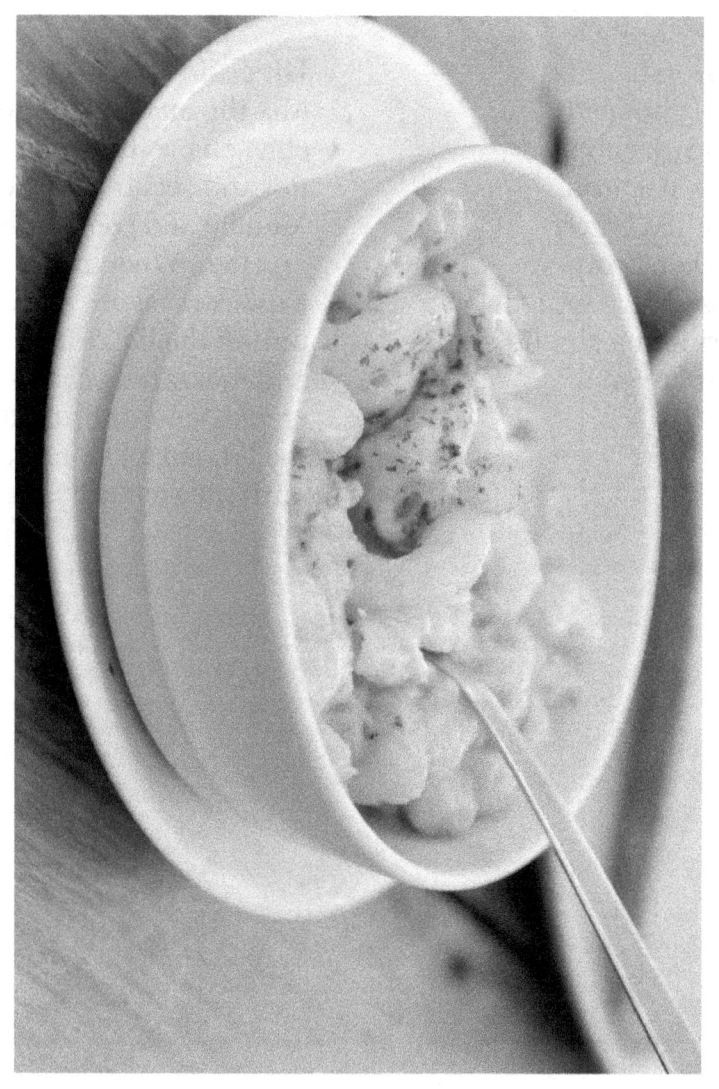

Green Goddess Mac 'n' Cheese

Prep.Time: 20 minutes
Servings: 4

Ingredients:
2 cups kale, chopped
2 tbsp cilantro, chopped
16 oz elbow macaroni
3 tbsp unsalted butter
4 cups chicken broth
3 cups mozzarella, grated
½ cup Parmesan, shredded
½ cup sour cream

Directions:
Mix the macaroni, butter, and chicken broth in your Instant Pot and seal the lid. Select Manual and cook for 4 minutes on High. When ready, perform a quick pressure release and unlock the lid. Stir in Parmesan and mozzarella cheeses, sour cream, kale, and cilantro. Put the lid and let sit for 5 minutes until the kale wilts. Serve.

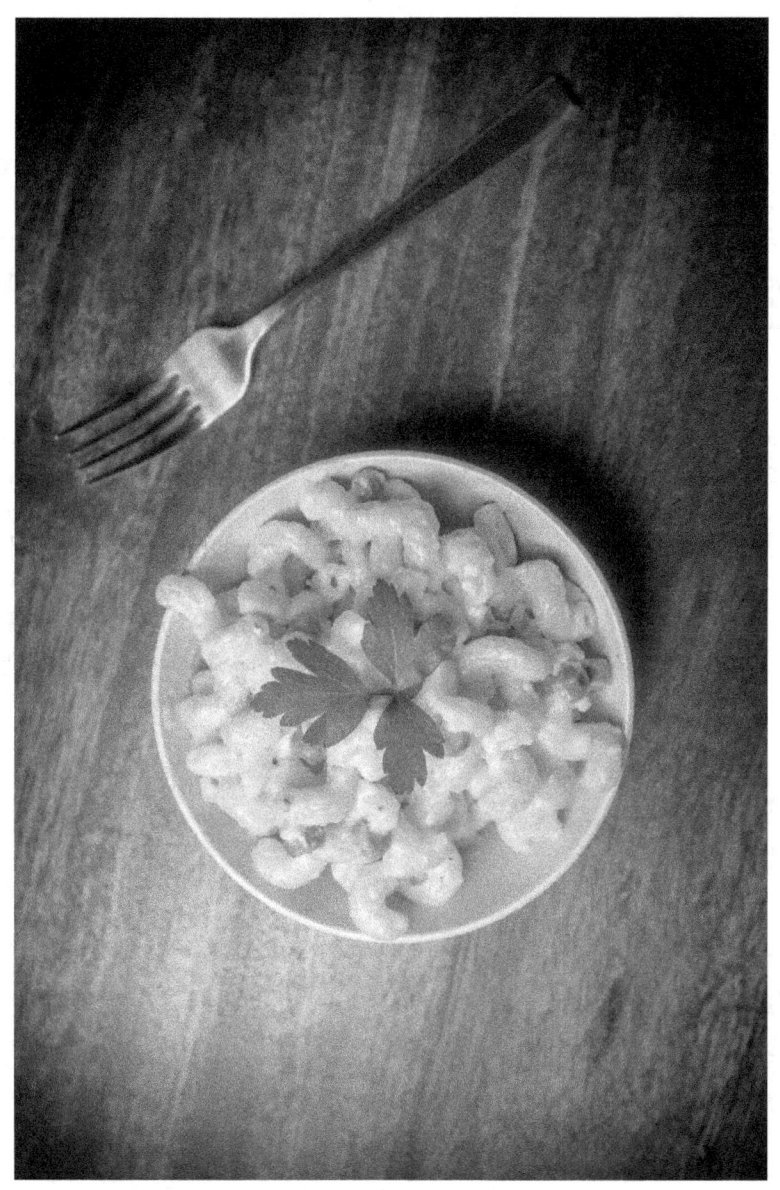

Chicken & Broccoli Fettuccine Alfredo

Prep.Time: 15 minutes
Servings: 2

Ingredients:
1 cup cooked chicken breasts, chopped
1 cup broccoli florets
8 oz fettuccine, halved
1 tsp chicken seasoning
1 jar (15 oz) Alfredo sauce
Salt and pepper to taste
1 tbsp parsley, chopped
1 tbsp Parmesan, grated

Directions:
Add 2 cups of water, fettuccine, and chicken seasoning to your Instant Pot. Place a steamer basket on top and add in the broccoli. Seal the lid, select Manual, and cook for 3 minutes on High. Once over, perform a quick pressure release. Drain the pasta and set aside. In a bowl, place Alfredo sauce, broccoli, parsley, and cooked chicken. Add in the pasta and mix to combine. Season with salt and pepper. Serve topped with Parmesan cheese.

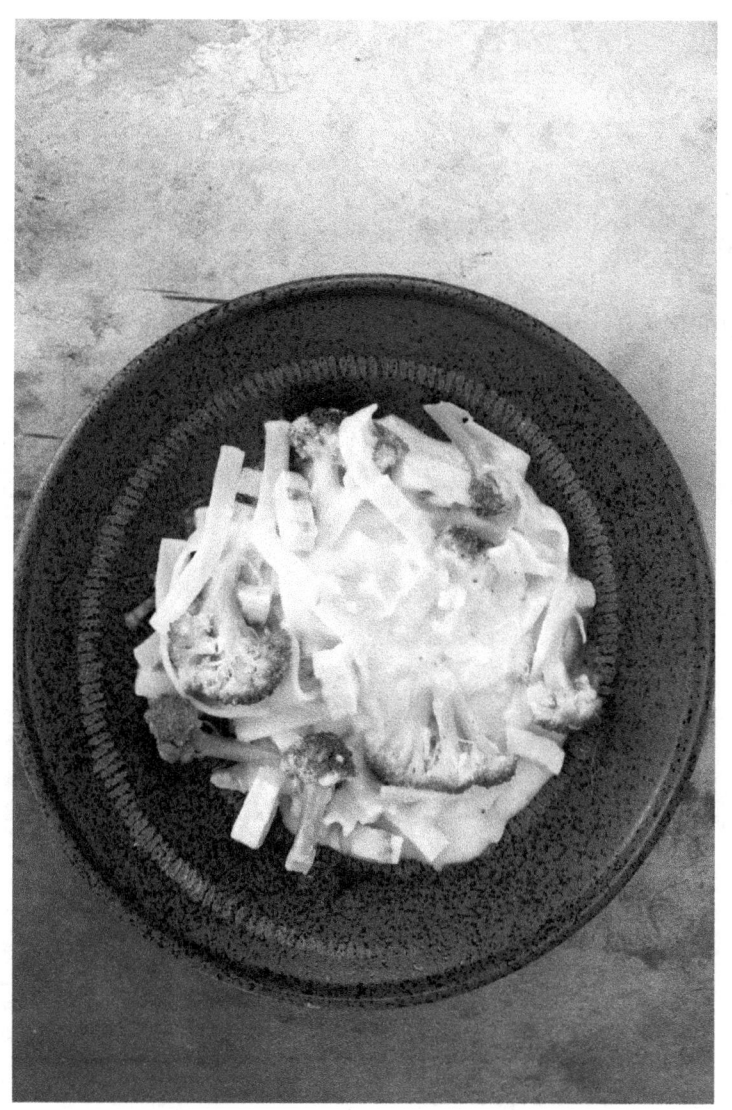

Easy Brown Rice with Sunflower Seeds

Prep.Time: 30 minutes
Servings: 6

Ingredients:
1 tbsp toasted sunflower seeds
1 ½ cups brown rice
3 cups chicken broth
2 tsp lemon juice
2 tsp olive oil
Salt and pepper to taste

Directions:
Add broth and brown rice. Season with salt and black pepper. Seal the lid, press Manual, and cook on High for 15 minutes. Release the pressure quickly. Do not open the lid for 5 minutes. Use a fork to fluff rice. Add lemon juice, sunflower seeds, and a drizzle of olive oil and serve.

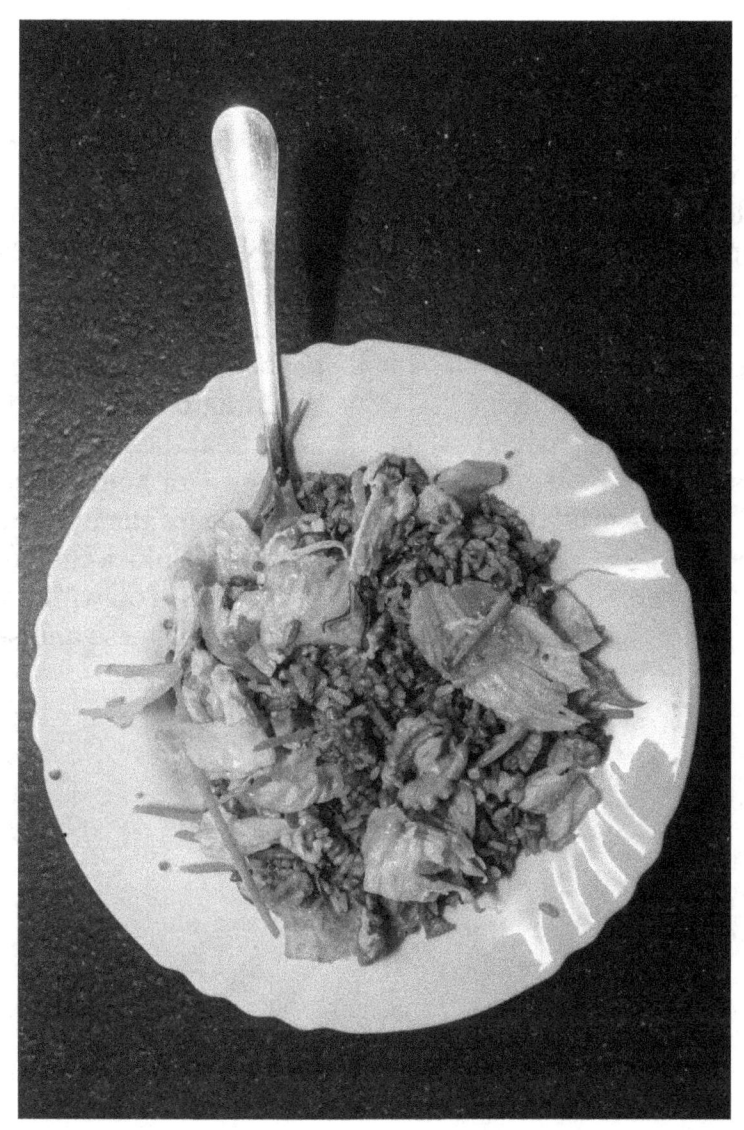

Spicy Linguine with Cherry Tomato & Basil

Prep.Time: 25 minutes
Servings: 4

Ingredients:
2 tbsp olive oil
1 small onion, diced
2 garlic cloves, minced
1 cup cherry tomatoes, halved
1 ½ cups vegetable stock
¼ cup julienned basil leaves
Salt and pepper to taste
¼ tsp red chili flakes
1 lb linguine noodles, halved
2 tbsp basil leaves
½ cup Parmesan, grated

Directions:
Warm oil on Sauté. Add onion and Sauté for 2 minutes until soft. Mix garlic and tomatoes and Sauté for 4 minutes. Add vegetable stock, salt, julienned basil, red chili flakes, and pepper to the pot. Add linguine to the tomato mixture until covered. Seal the lid. Cook on High Pressure for 5 minutes. Naturally release the pressure for 10 minutes. Unlock the lid. Divide into plates. Top with basil and Parmesan cheese and serve.

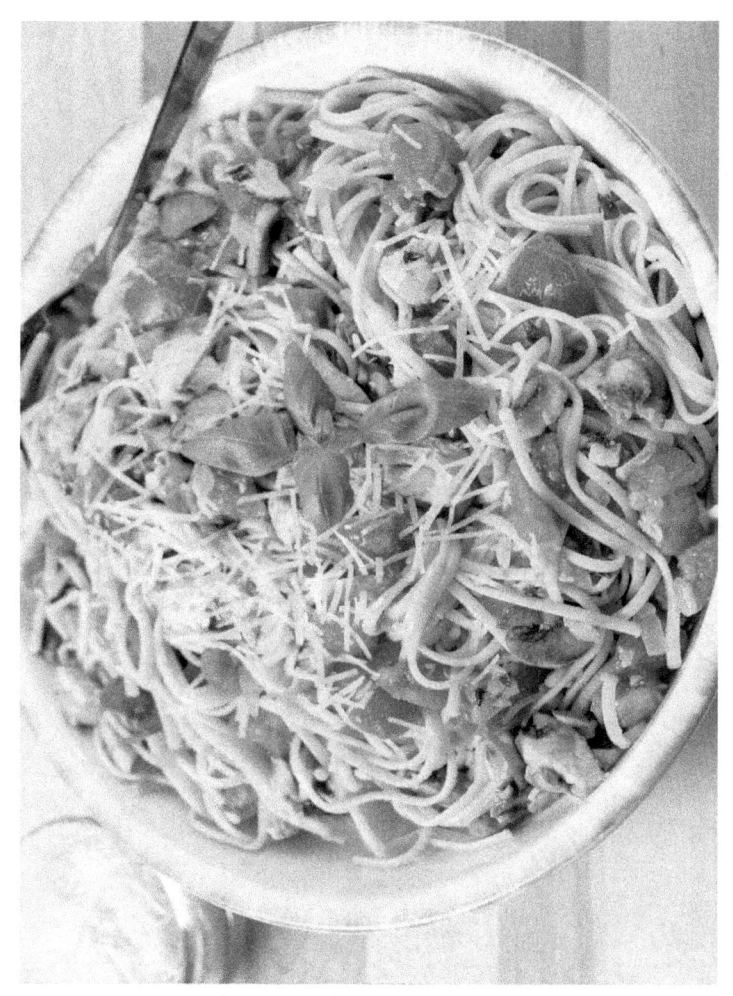

Chapter 9 Dinner

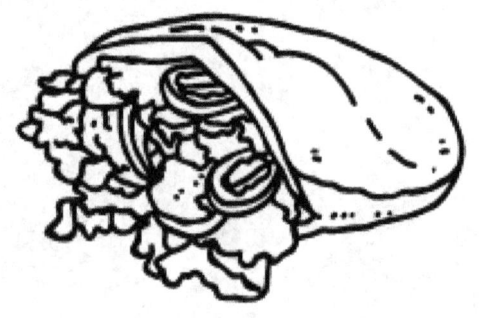

Butternut Squash with Rice & Feta

Prep.Time: 30 minutes
Servings: 4

Ingredients:
2 cups vegetable broth
1 lb butternut squash, sliced
2 tbsp melted butter
Salt and pepper to taste
1 cup feta cheese, cubed
1 tbsp coconut aminos
2 tsp arrowroot starch
1 cup jasmine rice, cooked

Directions:
Pour the rice and broth into the pot and stir to combine. In a bowl, toss butternut squash with 1 tbsp of melted butter and season with salt and black pepper. Mix in the pot with the rice. In another bowl, mix the remaining butter, water, and coconut aminos. Toss feta in the mixture, add the arrowroot starch, and toss again to combine well. Transfer to a greased baking dish. Lay a trivet over the rice butternut squash and place the baking dish on the trivet. Seal the lid and cook on High for 15 minutes. Do a quick pressure release. Fluff the rice with a fork and serve with feta cheese.

Avocado & Cherry Tomato Jasmine Rice

Prep.Time: 30 minutes
Servings: 6

Ingredients:
2 avocados, chopped
½ lb cherry tomatoes, halved
2 cups jasmine rice
2 tsp olive oil
½ tsp salt
2 tbsp cilantro, chopped

Directions:
Place the rice, 2 cups water, olive oil, and salt in your Instant Pot and stir. Seal the lid, select Manual, and cook for 4 minutes on High pressure. Once done, allow a pressure release for 10 minutes and unlock the lid. Using a fork, fluff the rice and add in avocados and cherry tomatoes. Top with cilantro and serve.

Date & Apple Risotto

Prep.Time: 30 minutes
Servings: 4

Ingredients:
1 tbsp butter
1 ½ cups Arborio rice
1/3 cup brown sugar
2 apples, cored and sliced
1 cup apple juice
2 cups milk
1 ½ tsp cinnamon powder
½ cup dates, pitted

Directions:
Melt butter in your Instant Pot on Sauté and place in rice; cook for 1-2 minutes. Stir in brown sugar, apples, apple juice, milk, and cinnamon. Seal the lid, select Manual, and cook for 6 minutes on High pressure. Once done, allow a natural release for 6 minutes and unlock the lid. Mix in dates and cover with the lid. Let sit for 5 minutes.

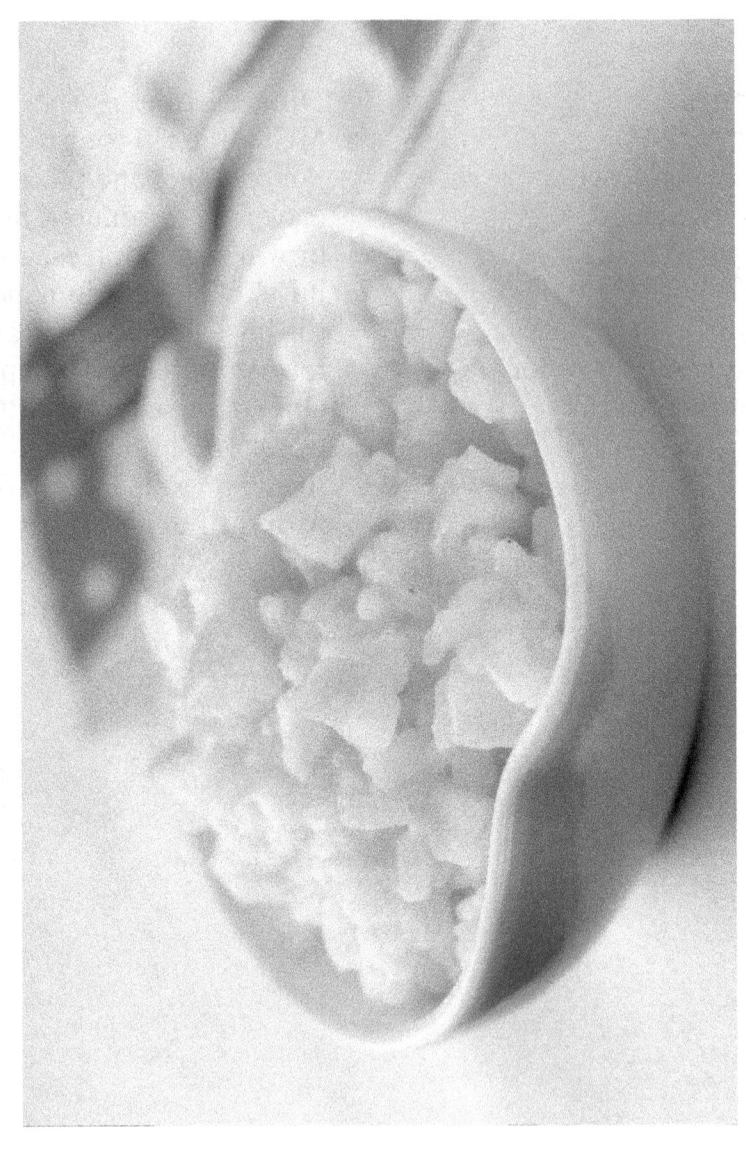

Butternut Squash & Cheese Risotto

Prep.Time: 45 minutes
Servings: 4

Ingredients:
½ lb butternut squash, cubed
3 tbsp olive oil
2 cloves garlic, minced
1 yellow onion, chopped
2 cups arborio rice
4 cups chicken stock
½ cup pumpkin puree
1 tsp thyme, chopped
½ tsp nutmeg
½ tsp ginger, grated
½ tsp cinnamon
½ cup heavy cream
Salt and pepper to taste
¼ cup shaved Parmesan

Directions:
Preheat the oven to 360°F. Spread the squash cubes on a baking tray and drizzle with olive oil. Roast for 20 minutes until tender. Warm oil in your Instant Pot on Sauté and add garlic and onion; cook for 3 minutes. Stir in rice, stock, pumpkin puree, thyme, nutmeg, ginger, and cinnamon. Seal the lid, select Manual, and cook for 10 minutes on High. When done, perform a quick pressure release. Mix in heavy cream, salt, and pepper. Top with pumpkin cubes and Parmesan shaves and serve.

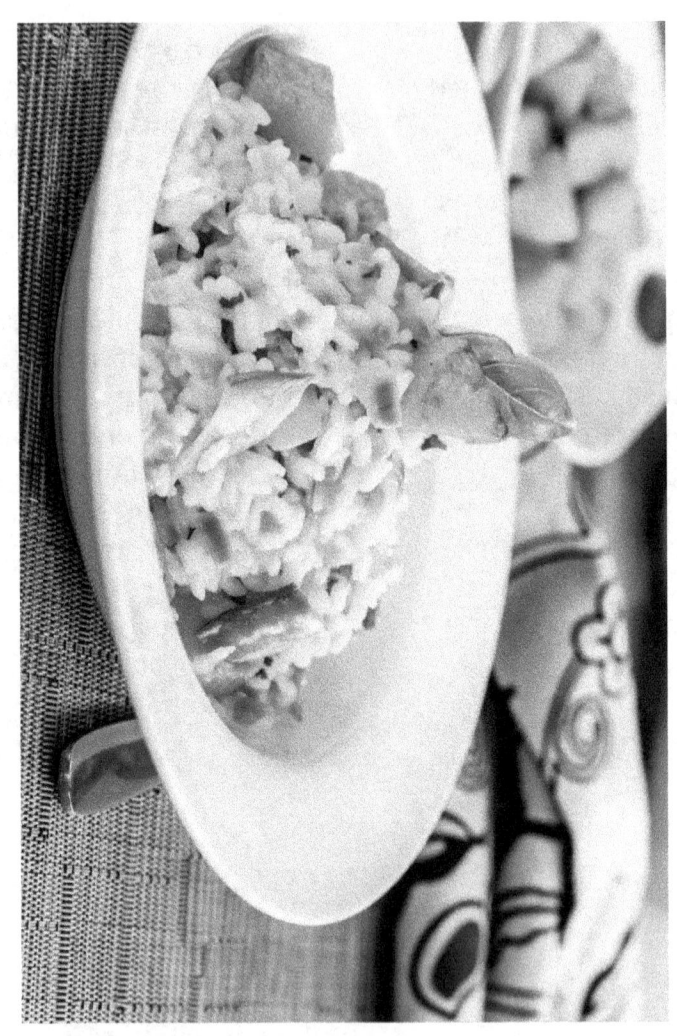

Spring Risotto

Prep.Time: 40 minutes
Servings: 6

Ingredients:
3 tbsp Pecorino Romano cheese, shredded
½ cup green peas
1 cup baby spinach
2 tbsp olive oil
2 spring onions, chopped
1 ½ cups arborio rice
3 ½ cups chicken stock
Salt and pepper to taste

Directions:
Warm olive oil in your Instant Pot on Sauté. Add spring onions and cook for 3 minutes. Pour in rice and stock. Seal the lid and cook for 15 minutes on Manual. Once done, allow a pressure release for 10 minutes and unlock the lid. Adjust the seasoning with salt and pepper. Mix in green peas and spinach and cover with the lid. Let sit for 5 minutes until everything is heated through. Top with Pecorino Romano cheese and serve.

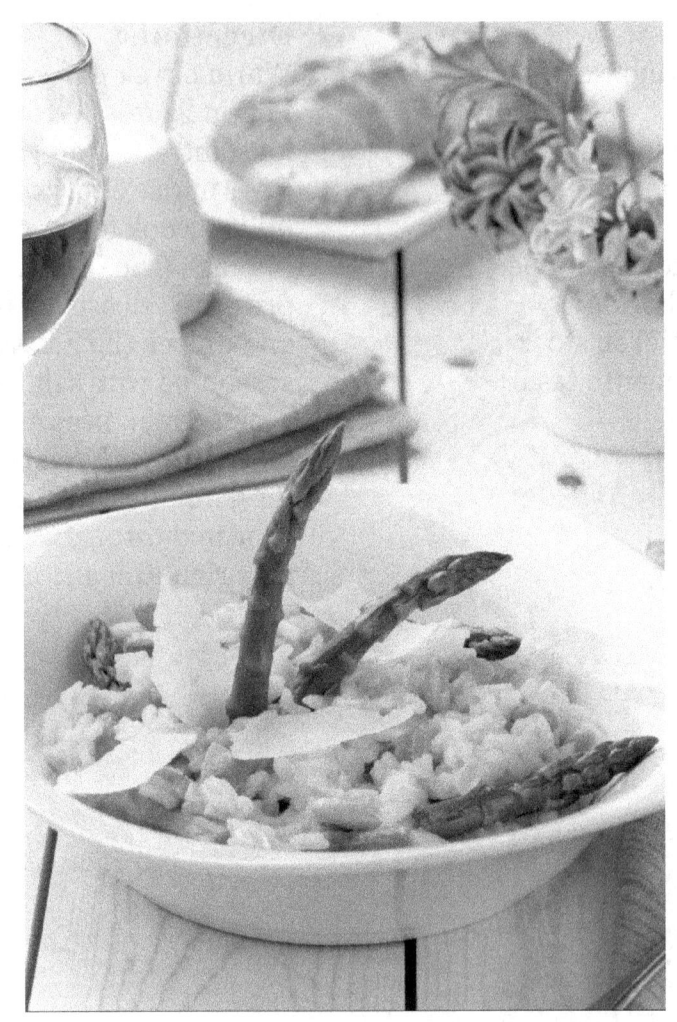

Arroz con Pollo

Prep.Time: 40 minutes
Servings: 4

Ingredients:
2 tbsp olive oil
1 sweet onion, diced
2 garlic cloves, minced
1 lb boneless chicken thighs
Salt and pepper to taste
½ tsp chili powder
2 carrots, diced
1 cup white jasmine rice
1 ½ cups chicken stock
½ tsp Mexican oregano

Directions:
Warm olive oil in your Instant Pot on Sauté. Add in onion and garlic and cook until fragrant, about 3 minutes. Stir in chicken, salt, and pepper and cook for 5 minutes more. Mix in carrots, rice, chili powder, chicken stock, and oregano. Seal the lid, select Manual, and cook for 10 minutes on High pressure. Once done, allow a pressure release for 10 minutes and unlock the lid. Fluff the rice.

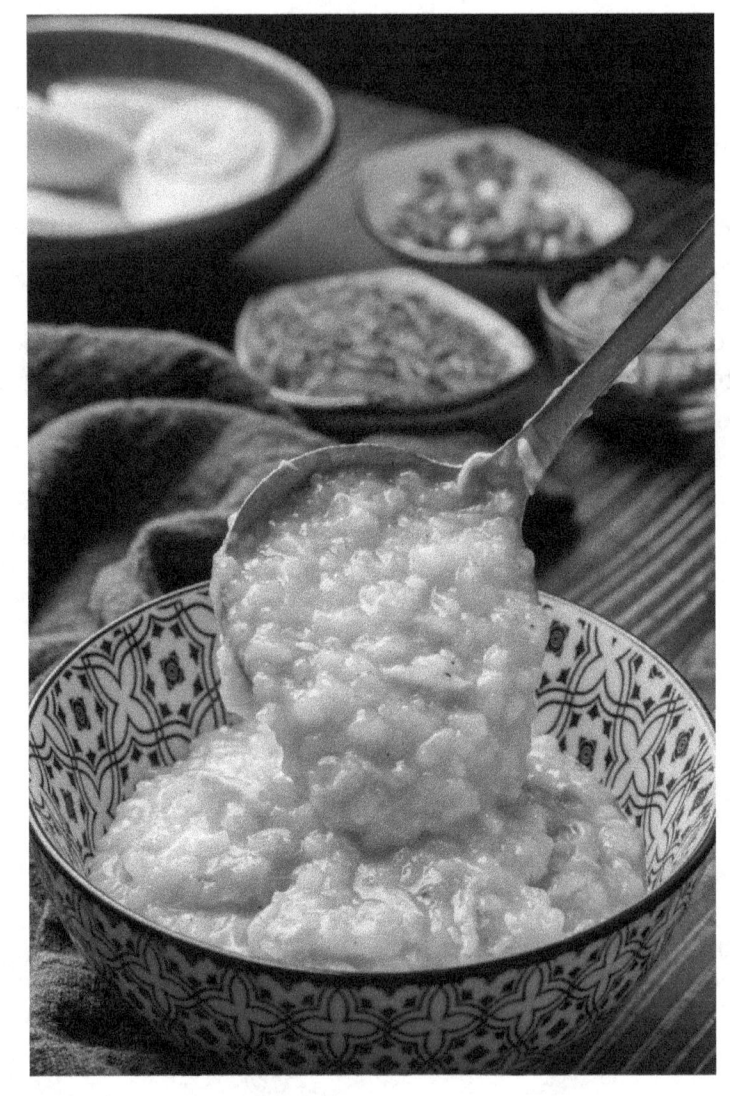

Chicken & Broccoli Rice

Prep.Time: 40 minutes
Servings: 4

Ingredients:
1 red chili, finely chopped
2 tbsp butter
1 lb chicken breasts, sliced
1 onion, chopped
2 cloves garlic, minced
Salt and pepper to taste
1 cup long-grain rice
2 cups chicken broth
10 oz broccoli florets
2 tbsp cilantro, chopped

Directions:
Melt butter in your Instant Pot on Sauté and add chicken, onion, red chili, garlic, salt, and pepper; cook for 5 minutes, stirring often. Stir in rice, chicken broth, milk, and broccoli. Seal the lid, select Manual, and cook for 15 minutes on High. When ready, allow a natural release for 10 minutes. Sprinkle with cilantro and serve.

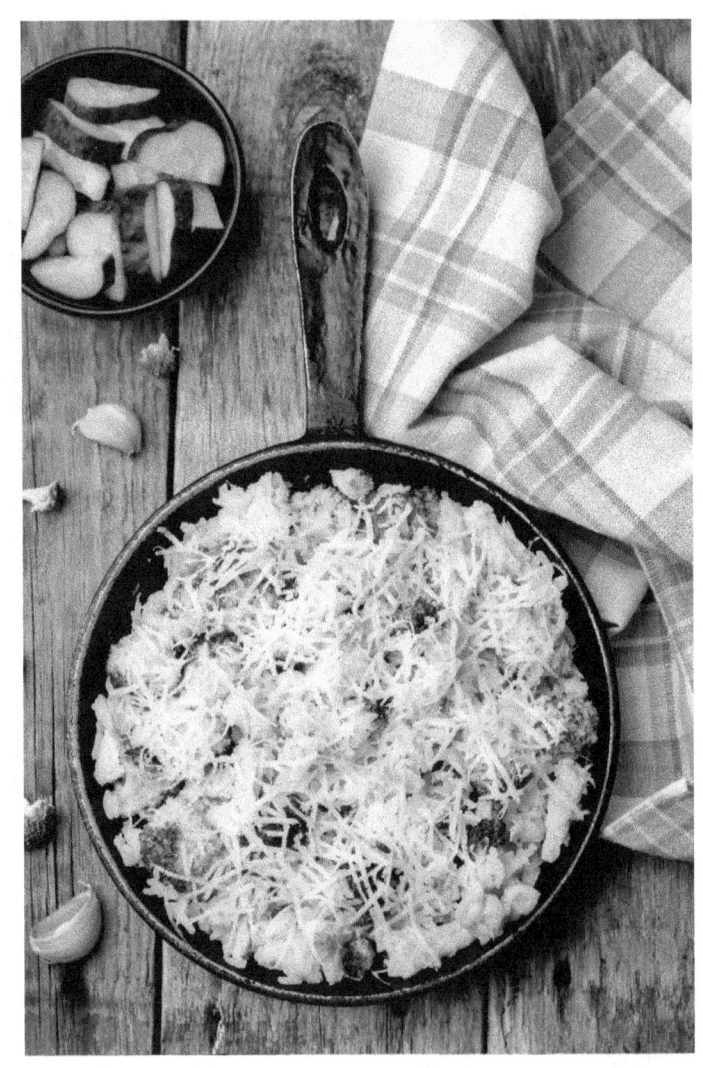

Hawaiian Rice

Prep.Time: 30 minutes
Servings: 4

Ingredients:
2 tsp olive oil
1 ½ cups coconut water
1 cup jasmine rice
2 green onions, sliced
½ pineapple, and chopped
Salt to taste
¼ tsp red pepper flakes

Directions:
Stir olive oil, water, rice, pineapple, and salt in your Instant Pot. Seal the lid, select Manual, and cook for 10 minutes on low pressure. Once over, allow a natural release for 10 minutes, then a quick pressure release. Carefully unlock the lid. Using a fork, fluff the rice. Scatter with green onions and red pepper flakes and serve.

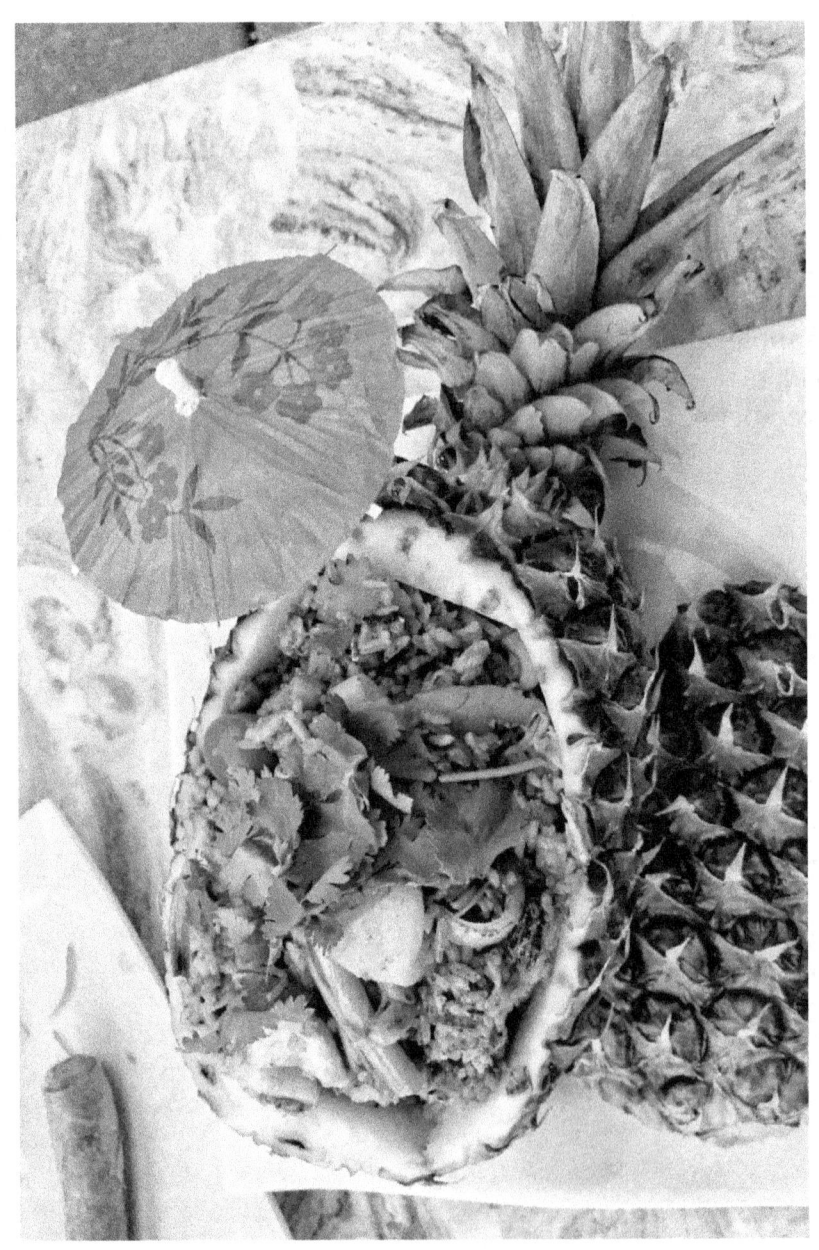

Index Recipes

A

Arroz con Pollo — 101
Avocado & Cherry Tomato Jasmine Rice — 94
Avocado Mousse with Chocolate — 74

B

Bacon, Cheese & Avocado Mug Cakes — 14
Baked Cod with Parmesan and Almonds — 54
Baked Haddock with Cheesy Topping — 52
Baked Pork Sausage with Vegetables — 40
Barbecued Pork Chops — 46
Basil Spinach & Zucchini Lasagna — 60
Butternut Squash & Cheese Risotto — 97
Butternut Squash with Rice & Feta — 93

C

Caramelized Onion & Cream Cheese Spread — 66
Cauli Rice Arancini — 62
Charred Broccoli with Tamarind Sauce — 36
Chicken, Avocado & Egg Bowls — 24
Chicken & Broccoli Fettuccine Alfredo — 86
Chicken & Broccoli Rice — 103
Chocolate Mousse Pots with Blackberries — 69
Citrus Pork with Cabbage & Tomatoes — 39
Coconut Avocado Tart — 29

D

Dark Chocolate Brownies — 70
Date & Apple Risotto — 95
Delicious Mushroom Pie — 32

E

Easy Brown Rice with Sunflower Seeds — 88

F

Favorite Peanut Butter Mousse — 72
Fiery Shrimp Cocktail Salad — 22
Flaxseed Toasts with Avocado Paté — 64

G

Greek Sea Bass with Olive Sauce --------------------------------- 56
Green Goddess Mac 'n' Cheese ---------------------------------- 84

H

Ham & Cheese Keto Sandwiches ---------------------------------- 9
Hawaiian Rice -- 105
Herb Pork Chops with Cranberry Sauce ------------------------- 44
Hot Broccoli Rabe --- 30

M

Maple Tahini Straws --- 59
Marinara Turkey Linguine -------------------------------------- 79
Mascarpone Cream Mousse --------------------------------------- 76
Mediterranean Artichoke Salad --------------------------------- 19
Mustard Macaroni & Cheese ------------------------------------- 82

P

Parmesan Shrimp Scampi Pizza ---------------------------------- 49
Pasta Tortiglioni with Beef & Black Beans --------------------- 80
Pork Chops with Basil-Tomato Sauce ---------------------------- 42
Pumpkin & Zucchini Bread -------------------------------------- 16

Q

Quick Tuna Omelet --- 50

S

Savory Waffles with Cheese & Tomato --------------------------- 10
Spicy Linguine with Cherry Tomato & Basil --------------------- 90
Spinach Salad with Pancetta & Mustard ------------------------- 26
Spring Risotto -- 99

T

Turkey Bacon & Turnip Salad ----------------------------------- 20

V

Vegetable Biryani --- 34

Z

Zesty Zucchini Bread with Nuts -------------------------------- 12

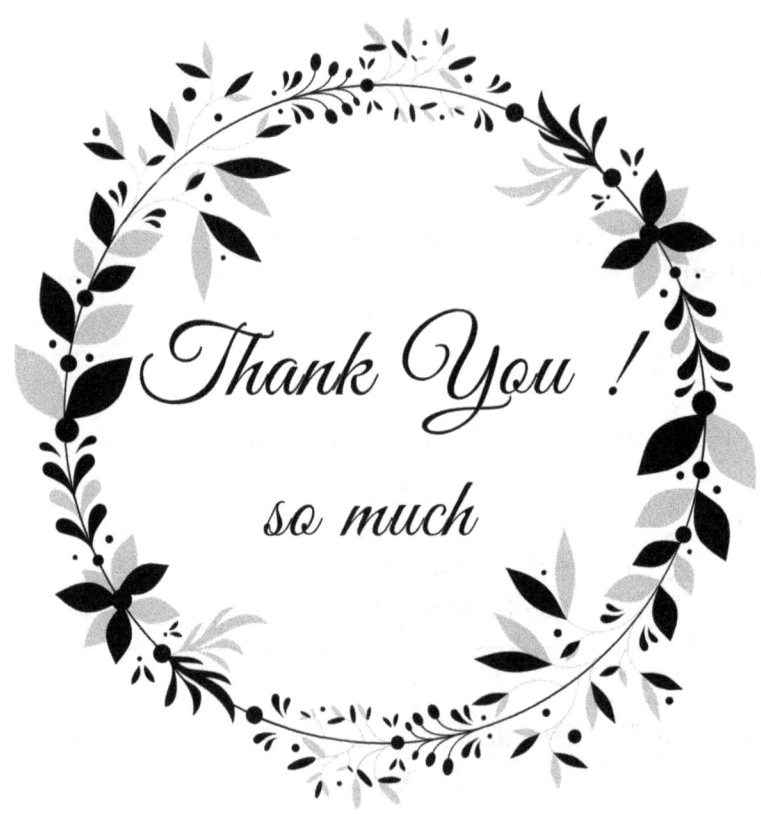

CPSIA information can be obtained
at www.ICGtesting.com
Printed in the USA
BVHW090331220621
610126BV00012B/2772